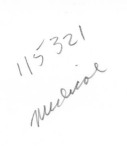

Timebomb

Timebomb

The Global Epidemic of Multi-Drug-Resistant Tuberculosis

Lee B. Reichman, M.D., M.P.H.
with Janice Hopkins Tanne

McGraw-Hill
New York   Chicago   San Francisco
Lisbon   London   Madrid   Mexico City   Milan
New Delhi   San Juan   Seoul   Singapore
Sydney   Toronto

McGraw-Hill

A Division of The McGraw-Hill Companies

Reichman, Lee B.
   Timebomb: the global epidemic of multi-drug resistant tuberculosis /
by Lee B. Reichman & Janice Hopkins Tanne.
      p.   cm.
      ISBN 0-07-135924-9
1. Tuberculosis—Popular works. 2. Multidrug resistance—Popular works.
   I. Tanne, Janice Hopkins. II. Title

RC312 .R454 2001
614.5'42 — dc21   2001034523

1 2 3 4 5 6 7 8 9 0   AGM/AGM   0 7 6 5 4 3 2 1

ISBN 0-07-135924-9

Printed and bound by Quebecor/Martinsburg.

 This book is printed on recycled, acid-free paper containing a minimum of 50% recycled de-inked fiber.

In memory of Julia M. Jones, MD, who passed on to me a small bit of her dedication, commitment, and passion relating to fighting tuberculosis,

and

To that brave, anonymous army who have devoted their careers, their health, and even their lives to the control of tuberculosis in often frustrating circumstances, when it was nobody's priority.

Lee B. Reichman

Contents

Preface

In the early 1990s, the United States was hit with an unprecedented epidemic of tuberculosis. The epicenter was in New York City, but cases rose nationally. At the time, I was president of the American Lung Association, and as spokesperson for this venerable voluntary health agency with its historical interest and involvement in this disease, I was deluged with calls from journalists, including Janice Hopkins Tanne. The city was terrified. This wasn't the ordinary kind of tuberculosis, which we've known how to cure for 50 years. This strain shrugged off most of the antibiotics we could throw at it. Ultimately, thanks to heroic efforts by the city's health department, headed by Dr. Margaret Hamburg — efforts aided by the Centers for Disease Control in Atlanta and the American Lung Association — the deadly outbreak was brought under control. The cost was $1 billion in excess health expenditures. How many cases of tuberculosis were involved?

When people hear the word "epidemic," they think, "Thousands dead! Bodies in the streets! Black Death! Ebola!" To public health experts, an epidemic is many more cases of a disease than they would otherwise expect. The number of tuberculosis cases in the United States and most of the industrialized world had been decreasing even before TB drugs were introduced in the 1940s, and cases were expected to continue falling. But funding was cut, beginning in the early 1970s. The years of success turned to failure. The ominous rise began in New York in 1979, and by 1985 TB cases were rising across the United States. By the end of the 1980s, New York had a full-blown epidemic. People are astonished to learn that in New York there were never more than 450 patients with active multi-drug-resistant tuberculosis at any one time. The entire epidemic involved fewer than 4000 cases per year at its height, between 1989 and 1992. Nevertheless, this was a major epidemic. These patients could infect family, friends, neighbors, coworkers, hospital staff members, and sometimes even casual contacts—people who breathed the same air.

To the ordinary person, 450 cases of multi-drug-resistant TB in a big city seems like a "so what" number. To a public health expert, it is a number that sends shivers up the spine.

You get tuberculosis by *breathing.* It is an airborne disease. Tuberculosis is expensive to treat, because finding cases requires relentless and discreet public health detection. Treatment means the patient must take four or more antibiotics for at least 6 months, preferably under the direct observation of dedicated health workers. All this requires backup: a reliable supply of effective drugs, good laboratories, and government commitment. New York was fortunate: It had an extraordinary health commissioner in Hamburg, and it had support from city, state, and federal authorities. And the country was rich enough to deal with the danger to public health.

The cost of controlling this outbreak of TB was "phenomenal," according to a report the New York City team[1] published in the *New England Journal of Medicine:* Public health structures and institutions that had been allowed to waste away had to be rebuilt. Health department personnel to find patients had to be hired. The closed and shuttered chest clinics had to be reopened. Free drugs had to be provided to cure patients. Hospitals and prisons had to be renovated so that people with active TB would not endanger others. Expert help had to be obtained to record and track TB patients so that they did not fall through the cracks. Treatment of latent infection had to be provided to people who had been infected by those with active tuberculosis.

After all was said and done, this $1 billion in excess health-care costs over a period of 2 or 3 years was successfully spent, and the New York City epidemic was contained. But, ominously, the tuberculosis timebomb still lurks in hot spots around the globe, all of them only hours away from our doorsteps in the United States and other industrialized countries. Tuberculosis has not gone away, although once again it has strayed far from the public mind in prosperous nations. Fully one-third of the world's population is infected with latent tuberculosis—2 billion people, including at least 15 million Americans. And 10 percent of those infected will develop active, usually infectious, TB during their lifetimes.

The global epidemic is getting worse every year. The number of people with active TB is growing: According to the World Health Organization, there were 8.4 million new cases in 1999 (the last year for which we have statistics), up from 8 million the year before.[2] Each year, 2 to 3 million people die from tuberculosis, more than from any other single infection, despite the fact that the disease in its most common form is entirely preventable and treatable. People who are infected with HIV (the virus that causes AIDS) are uniquely susceptible to TB; fully treatable TB remains the leading cause of death worldwide among AIDS patients.

More people are dying of tuberculosis today than ever before in history.

Worse yet, years of neglect and mismanagement have created multi-drug-resistant strains of TB, which are curable only at enormous cost and effort when they can be cured at all. While the Third World struggles to cope with ordinary TB and other pressing public health issues and the industrialized nations assume that TB is a thing of the past that they can safely ignore, this almost incurable form of tuberculosis is quickly spreading from Russia and other "TB hot spots" to the rest of the world. Drug-resistant TB strains from the former Soviet Union have already appeared in several parts of the United States. TB rates are rising in many Western European countries, and London already has a TB epidemic.

Some 50 million people visit the United States each year. An additional 660,000 come as legal immigrants, and it is estimated from the most recent census that there are 7.1 to 9 million illegal immigrants living in the nation.[3] Thanks to modern air travel, it takes only a day to reach the United States or other industrialized nations from anywhere in the world. Only people entering the United States as permanent immigrants are screened for TB; other Western nations do even less screening. No one knows how many illegal immigrants arrive with TB. We do know that almost half of the active cases of TB in the United States, 46 percent, occur in people born outside the country; the situation is similar in other Western countries.

Looking at this international tuberculosis timebomb, in 1993, as the recent New York (and U.S.) epidemic was being brought under control with great effort, Janice and I proposed a book about the looming threat. A well-connected literary agent took the idea to at least 30 of the world's leading publishers. They all turned it down.

However, the acquisitions editor at one major publisher did call me. She was a middle-class, university-educated, white woman in her early thirties. She said that she had just learned from a positive tuberculin skin test that she had been infected with tuberculosis. She asked me what she should do. Was she ill? Could she infect her family, friends, and colleagues? Should she take antibiotics? Which ones? Could her tuberculosis be resistant to antibiotics, maybe incurable?

I responded by giving her my best professional advice, and then, encouraged by her questions, I asked whether she would like us to write the book, to tell people about this ubiquitous threat. "Oh, no," she said. "People wouldn't be interested."

This middle-class woman had just had a positive skin test, which meant that she had been infected with tuberculosis, and she was essentially telling us that only poor people and minorities get TB and that the people who buy books wouldn't be interested. This is the classic problem that those of us who work with TB encounter all the time. Though it is first among the world's infectious killers, TB has an image problem. It is a plague—alas, just like AIDS—that ordinary, middle-class people think they will never get, or ever be exposed to.

The tuberculosis crisis is rapidly getting worse, even as I write these words. Russia has created a disastrous TB epidemic in its prisons and is spreading it through the release of hundreds of thousands of prisoners each year. Furthermore, misplaced Russian nationalism (medical jingoism) is preventing them from joining the global medical community in using internationally accepted, scientifically proven (evidence-based) treatment for TB. AIDS cases are increasing faster in Russia than anywhere else in the world, and AIDS and TB are like gasoline and a match. Besides Russia, the World Health Organization has identified 21 other TB hot spots around the world. The threat is at our doorstep, and we can no longer ignore it. The timebomb is about to explode, and we are not ready.

We have no new diagnostic tests for tuberculosis, no new drugs, no magic cures. Even in the high-tech medical centers of the United States and other industrialized countries, doctors use nineteenth-century diagnostic methods and 30- to 50-year-old treatments—because there are no others—for a disease that is running way ahead of us. Until very recently, there was no interest in this crisis from anybody except the few physicians, nurses, and health-care workers who treat tuberculosis daily. But things are beginning to change.

Tuberculosis has probably been with us since the invention of agriculture. But it can be stopped. We are at a critical juncture in our battle against this deadly foe. Left unchecked, it will, without question, continue to gain momentum in its new, incurable, airborne form, but there is hope that this threat is finally being recognized. In a few circles at least, there are signs of burgeoning interest in building the political will and international cooperation that are needed if we are to find new diagnostic methods, drugs, and vaccines.

Tuberculosis remains an ancient disease that has killed more people worldwide than any other single infection in human history. Paradoxically, although effective drugs and other interventions have been available for 50 years, there has been an embarrassingly meager effort to control the disease. We have the tools and we have not used them.

This book describes the changing response of society to this devastating illness in the past few years. Now, governments and businesses are beginning to consider tuberculosis as an economic and tourism problem, not merely a social or health problem affecting mostly the poor. At the same time, a number of high-profile, but untraditional, individuals and organizations interested in public health have become involved, some even passionately so.

Although such new players have joined the fight, giving hope that we may win our long struggle against TB, cases and deaths have actually increased. Today we face a growing international threat from the most serious form of the disease—multi-drug-resistant TB. As this book will show, progress against TB is slow and may be fatally detoured by developments in Russia.

While the new high profile of tuberculosis is well deserved, we cannot forget the legions of workers, both professional and nonprofessional, who have devoted their careers, their health, and even their lives to the control of tuberculosis in often frustrating circumstances, when it was nobody's priority. These dedicated workers essentially "kept the lid on" until political will began to attack the TB problem, bringing new players, new funds, and new successes.

This book is written in a salute to that brave, anonymous army. If TB is ultimately controlled and even eliminated, those who toiled in tuberculosis control when it was merely frustrating and not "sexy" laid the foundation for later progress and success.

We hope that this book will help to sound the alarm and contribute to those efforts that will relegate this preventable, treatable, curable disease to the history books where it belongs. In our global society, we must realize that to control tuberculosis anywhere, we must control tuberculosis everywhere.

Please visit us at our Web site, www.tbtimebomb.com, for continuing updates on the epidemic.

Lee B. Reichman, M.D., M.P.H

Acknowledgments

I started as an academic lung physician with a prime interest in tuberculosis, a neglected disease that was not a popular subject for study. Therefore, I thank some of the giants in this field whose guidance and inspiration allowed me to continue and advance: Professors George Comstock and Gerry Baum, and Drs. Phyllis Edwards and Annik Rouillon.

As chief of a pulmonary division working on an unpopular disease at an academic medical center, I acknowledge support from above to continue in my sometimes unconventional ways, and so I thank the administration of The University of Medicine and Dentistry of New Jersey, my past dean at the New Jersey Medical School, Dr. Ruy Lourenco, Vice Dean Dr. Tony Garro, and my past department chairs, Drs. Francis P. Chinard, Carroll M. Leevy, and Waldemar G. (Buzz) Johanson. They all supported—often cheerfully—my aspirations and ambitions.

The agencies I have worked with have also supported me and my ideas. John Garrison and Nereida Torres of the American Lung Association always helped me look good, and Fran DuMelle taught me advocacy and the proper, seminal role of a nongovernmental agency in creating and implementing public policy. The senior staff of the Centers for Disease Control and Prevention Tuberculosis Elimination Division—Drs. Kenneth Castro and his colleagues Carl Schiffelbein, John Seggerson, Dr. Rick O'Brien, Dr. Pattie Simone, Dr. Ida Onorato, Dr. Wanda Walton, and Kenneth L. Shilkret, the CDC assignee to New Jersey—have been good friends and colleagues and, for the most part, supported my ideas and programs.

My academic pursuits were aided by publication of the first scientific textbook on TB in 30 years (*Tuberculosis: A Comprehensive International Approach*), and I thank my co-editor, Dr. Earl Hershfield of the University of Manitoba, for his patience and energy.

Clearly, I was able to be involved in and to contribute to the fight against TB on the national and international level because my "day job" at the New Jersey Medical School Pulmonary Division since 1974 and, since 1993, at the New Jersey Medical School National Tuberculosis Center which has been run efficiently and effectively by an extraordinary staff. My thanks go especially to my close clinical associates, Drs. Reynard McDonald and Bonita Mangura, my colleague and deputy director Eileen C. Napolitano, program assistant Robin Dove, director of training and education Debra Kantor, nurse manager Lillian Pirog, and to my long-time secretary Jean Norwood.

***

Janice and I are grateful for the cooperation we have received from Ann Cohen, public relations director, and Lew Weinstein, president, and the entire staff of the Public Health Research Insitute; from Oksana I. Ponomarenko of the PHRI Moscow office; from Yuriy Longinov, a skilled translator based in Moscow; from Rachel Fisher Abram in New York, a careful and thorough researcher; and from Alfred Paspe, user support specialist at the New Jersey Medical School, and Michael Jesser of By Design, for their skill in Web design and electronic wizardry. We have been fortunate to have an enthusiastic and caring agent in Jane Dystel, and excellent, thorough editors at McGraw-Hill—Amy Murphy and Ruth Mannino. This book is better for their painstaking work.

Finally, I would like to acknowledge the patience, dedication, and support of my wife, Rose Reichman, and our children, Daniel Mark and Deborah Gar Reichman.

Lee B. Reichman

In addition to the many colleagues whose assistance to me and to Dr. Reichman has been acknowledged above, I would like to honor the shining example set by the late Dr. Jonathan Mann, a public health leader and AIDS crusader, who taught that health is a human right.

I offer my heartfelt thanks to my husband, Sol Tanne, for his unswerving and loving support throughout my long work on this book, and to our daughter, Duchess, for her assistance.

Janice Hopkins Tanne

1

Ebola with Wings

> "Tuberculosis is Ebola with wings."
>
> — *Richard Bumgarner, World Health Organization, 1993*

On September 2, 1998, a crowd of passengers in an air-conditioned departure lounge in Paris stirred restlessly, waiting for their flight from Charles De Gaulle Airport to John F. Kennedy Airport in New York. American tourists returning home were culture crammed and shopped out. Trendy young French people dressed in black leather, were planning for tourist adventures in New York's SoHo and Tribeca or visits to the Guggenheim and the Museum of Modern Art. French businesspeople, well tailored and trim, were equipped with cell phones and laptops. A handful of French families were perhaps planning to take their kids to the Grand Canyon or Disneyland or the White House. Travelers were on their way, via New York, to other destinations. These were just a few of the approximately 50 million international travelers who come to the United States every year.

One group of travelers in the departure lounge looked different. These people were a little bit shabby, and among themselves they spoke an unfamiliar language. It wasn't French or English or Spanish or German. It wasn't Dutch or a Scandinavian tongue. It was Ukrainian. They were immigrants, going to join a group of other Ukrainians who had already settled in the United States. Among them was a thin, pale man in his thirties. A younger woman, probably his wife, sat next to him. She looked anxious. The man looked ill. He coughed into his handkerchief.

The flight began boarding.[1] It was almost full, with nearly 300 passengers cheek by jowl, elbows bumping. The plane pulled away from the gate and taxied out onto the runway, where it sat, waiting for takeoff. The delay

dragged on for about 30 minutes, and the air grew stuffy, as fresh air circulation was not as good while the aircraft was on the ground as when it would
be when the plane was in the air. Finally the plane took off.

The flight was routine: seven and a half hours to JFK Airport in New
York, with the usual movies, meals, headsets, duty-free, strolls up and down
the aisle, lines for the toilets. The passenger in row 30, seat 5—the thin, pale
man who spoke Ukrainian—coughed the whole way. He did not look well.

Three days later, on September 5, the Ukrainian man—let's call him
Nikolay Ivanov—walked into a public health clinic in a small town in Erie
County, Pennsylvania, in the western part of the state. He knew he was ill.
He probably even knew what the illness was. After all, he'd had bouts of it
for 20 years and had been treated for it several times in Ukraine.

What he had was active tuberculosis. Although he did not know it that
day in Erie County, he was the index case, the first identified source of a
spreading infection that could become an epidemic. The source case, the
person from whom he had been infected with TB, is unknown and probably will never be identified. Every time Nikolay coughed, he unleashed millions and millions of tuberculosis bacteria that floated invisibly in the air
—millions and millions of bacteria that could infect anyone who breathed
them in.

In Bill Barry's small, cluttered cubicle in Harrisburg, the capital of
Pennsylvania, the phone rang. Barry, a senior public health adviser with the
Division of Tuberculosis Elimination of the Centers for Disease Control and
Prevention (CDC), had been on loan to the Tuberculosis Control Program
of the Pennsylvania Department of Health for many years. The public health
adviser program was started by the CDC during World War II to cope with
an epidemic of sexually transmitted diseases. Although public health advis-
ers are not doctors, they are usually more knowledgeable about communicable diseases than most doctors. Like detectives, they help state health
departments track disease patterns, looking for the source of an outbreak and
doing "contact tracing," or finding people who may have been infected by a
sick person. It is dedicated work, often in unpleasant neighborhoods, dealing with people who may not want to hear that they have been infected with
an unpopular disease and do not want to have someone coming daily to see
that they take their medicine. "It's tough work. It can be dangerous. These
people are public health heroes," said John Seggerson, associate director of
the CDC's Division of Tuberculosis Elimination.

The phone call meant that Barry was about to begin work on a potential outbreak of TB imported from Ukraine by that traveler on the flight from
Paris to New York. "The doctor at the clinic called and told me he suspected

tuberculosis. He made this preliminary diagnosis based on the man's symptoms," Barry said. That was in itself rather startling, because most American doctors are so unfamiliar with this old but now resurgent disease that they wouldn't recognize it if a TB patient coughed in their face. In Pennsylvania, there are only 3.7 cases of tuberculosis per 100,000 people, a blessedly low rate that is a tribute to Pennsylvania's effective public health department. In Ukraine, there are more than ten times as many cases—52.9 cases per 100,000.[2] Elsewhere in the former Soviet Union, particularly in the prisons, TB rates are a thousand times higher than they are in Pennsylvania.

The people of Pennsylvania were lucky that Nikolay was a legal immigrant, not an illegal immigrant or a tourist or business visitor to the United States. All documented (legal) immigrants to the United States over the age of 15 are required to produce a chest X-ray taken within the last 12 months that shows that they are free of active tuberculosis.[3] Immigration officials know the system isn't perfect. A prospective immigrant can easily buy the X-ray of a healthy person on the black market or submit the X-ray of a healthy friend or relative. Nevertheless, immigrants undergo more screening than people who simply visit the United States as tourists or for business.

Would-be immigrants who have X-rays showing active and infectious tuberculosis are called "Class A" and are forbidden entry to the United States. Class B1 immigrants have active TB but are not infectious (for example, because their TB affects bones or joints and can't be coughed out to cause infection). Class B2 immigrants have signs of old, inactive TB. All Class B immigrants are allowed into the United States, but they are informed that they must be further evaluated for tuberculosis when they arrive at their destination. State health departments are notified about all Class B immigrants and are expected to report back to the Division of Quarantine on their evaluation of the immigrant. Nikolay's chest X-ray, taken in Ukraine, had indeed been abnormal, showing signs of possible active tuberculosis. He was required to have a test of his sputum (called an acid-fast smear) in Ukraine. It was negative, showing no tuberculosis bacteria, so he was classified as a B1 immigrant—with TB, but noninfectious. However, the classification was made several months before he entered the United States.

At just about the same time as Nikolay walked into the health clinic complaining of feeling ill, the Pennsylvania Health Department was notified by the U.S. Immigration and Naturalization Service that his X-ray was suspicious for TB. "We received a 'refugee placement form,' as it's called, from the U.S. officials who had screened Nikolay in Ukraine long before he arrived in the United States. It was one of the times when the system worked," Barry explained. Though Nikolay had been considered noninfectious when he applied for a visa almost a year earlier, he was certainly sick and very likely infectious now, as the doctor at the public health clinic in western Pennsylvania could easily see.

The clinic doctor had Nikolay cough up sputum samples on September 5, 6, and 7. When the sputum was stained and examined under a microscope, all the samples were positive for the vicious little red bars of acid-fast bacilli, strongly suggesting that the man had active, infectious tuberculosis. The clinic doctor immediately started Nikolay on a five-drug regimen that he hoped would cure the tuberculosis: isoniazid, rifampin, pyrazinamide, ethambutol, and streptomycin. The doctor did not merely hand Nikolay a fistful of prescriptions. Nikolay had to take eight pills and one very painful injection every day. The health-care worker who gave the injection watched to see that Nikolay took all the pills. If a health-care worker just hands a prescription to a patient, there is no guarantee that the patient will fill the prescription and take the drugs for the months required to cure TB. Compliance with medication regimens is just as lax among investment bankers and doctors as among homeless alcoholics or newly arrived Ukrainians. The best way to cure the patient and protect the community is to deliver the pills to the patient and watch the patient take them. In Pennsylvania, with its excellent public health system, directly observed treatment of TB with antibiotics is available free of charge, but, unfortunately, many other states have not made as extensive a commitment to protecting their citizens from tuberculosis.

Bill Barry and the clinic doctor were concerned that Nikolay's TB might not be treatable with the standard drugs. Like the rest of the former Soviet Union, Ukraine is considered to be one of the world's hot spots for multi-drug-resistant tuberculosis. Multi-drug-resistant tuberculosis is defined by the World Health Organization and the International Union Against Tuberculosis and Lung Disease, the most important organizations dealing with TB worldwide, as tuberculosis that is resistant to the two strongest and most important TB drugs, isoniazid and rifampin. Unlike ordinary tuberculosis, whose 6-month treatment is arduous enough, multi-drug-resistant tuberculosis (MDR-TB) requires treatment for as long as 2 years with much more expensive drugs that often have unpleasant and harmful side effects such as hearing loss, stomach upsets, kidney damage, liver damage, dizziness, psychosis, and depression. In some cases, MDR-TB is completely incurable: Nothing kills the tuberculosis bacteria and the patient may die. Meanwhile, the dying patient can infect anyone who comes near him or her with the same incurable tuberculosis.

Just like ordinary tuberculosis, MDR-TB is spread through the air by coughing or sneezing—sometimes even by speaking, if the tuberculosis has infected the larynx.

Working with an interpreter, the Pennsylvania health department people interviewed Nikolay, their index case, and his family members. Nikolay said that he had had tuberculosis for more than 20 years, since he was an adolescent. He had been treated for it in 1976, 1985, and 1986, and again from 1992 to 1994. Had he received precisely the right drugs, in the right dosages, for the right length of time? It didn't seem likely. Even if he had received a good plan of treatment, it may well have been with poor-quality drugs that weren't absorbed well. Either way, there was a good chance that he had developed resistance to the standard TB drugs.

Working with Bill Barry, the clinic doctor in western Pennsylvania sent samples of Nikolay's sputum to three highly sophisticated reference laboratories: the Pennsylvania health department laboratory, the CDC laboratory in Atlanta, and the Wadsworth Laboratory (headed by Max Salfinger) of the New York State Health Department in Albany, a regional reference laboratory. (Reference laboratories are laboratories that check and confirm the results from other labs.) Barry asked the three laboratories to do tuberculosis drug sensitivity tests. It was the only way to know if Nikolay was getting the right drugs.

At these sophisticated labs, technicians must work in high-tech biosafety rooms for protection from infectious bacteria that may become airborne. There are four levels of biosafety labs. TB studies must be done in biosafety level 3 (BSL-3) labs if the technicians are doing basic research and dealing with large quantities of infectious organisms. For smaller studies such as those to determine the drugs to which Nikolay's tuberculosis was sensitive, a BSL of 2+ is adequate. That still means that for their own protection against these lethal organisms, technicians must wear government-certified respirators, that they can handle TB bacteria only in special cabinets with hoods that shield them against the bacteria, and that the lab must have negative air pressure. Negative air pressure means that the air pressure in the anteroom to the lab is lower than that in the common hall, and the air pressure in the lab itself is lower than that in the anteroom. Therefore, whenever a door is opened, air flows from the hall into the anteroom and from the anteroom into the lab and is then sent out through special filters that trap any TB bacteria. This ensures that no stray bacteria can flow in the reverse direction and escape from the lab into the common hall.

In each of the three reference labs, samples of Nikolay's sputum were transferred to culture dishes. Each culture dish contained a different antibiotic. If the TB bacteria grew in the presence of the antibiotic, that showed that they were resistant to that antibiotic and it would be useless in treating Nikolay. If the bacteria did not grow in the presence of the antibiotic, it showed that they were sensitive to that antibiotic. Thus, technicians could tell Barry and the clinic doctor which antibiotics killed the bacteria and therefore could be used to treat Nikolay. His sputum had to be tested against the nine antibiotics used to treat ordinary TB and multidrug-resistant TB.

The problem was that this would take a long time. The bacteria that cause pneumonia and other common infections such as strep throat double every 20 minutes, but TB bacteria are extremely slow to grow, taking 20 to 24 hours to double. It would be weeks, at best, before the labs could detect the drug sensitivity pattern of Nikolay's TB, weeks before Barry and the clinic doctor would know whether Nikolay, their index case, was getting the right drugs to cure his disease and protect the community.

Meanwhile, Nikolay's contacts in his Pennsylvania community had to be tested, and the airline crew and the 300 or so other passengers on Nikolay's flight had to be found and tested. There was nothing Barry or anyone else could do about people who might have strolled through the departure lounge at Charles De Gaulle Airport or stopped nearby for a glass of wine and a sandwich. Nor was there any way to find people who had been picking up their baggage from the same carousel or waiting in the same line for the immigration agent or the customs agent or crowded into the arrivals area where passengers meet family and friends. And who knew whom Nikolay had been in contact with on bus, train, or car as he traveled from New York City to western Pennsylvania? The one piece of good news was that the shorter the exposure time, the less likely it was that TB transmission had occurred. Although it is possible to be infected with TB after a very brief exposure, it usually takes days or weeks of exposure to a person with active TB to cause infection, and some people manage to avoid infection even then. It was unlikely, although not impossible, that someone who had had only brief contact with Nikolay could have been infected with his tuberculosis.

Barry was well aware of the risk of tuberculosis transmission on an airplane. Public health people knew of a flight attendant who had spread TB to many of the crew she usually worked with. In 1998 the World Health Organization declared that flights of more than 8 hours posed the risk of exposing passengers and crew to infectious tuberculosis.[4] The medical literature includes many examples. In a case reported in the *New England Journal of Medicine*, an Asian tourist infected at least six airline passengers while traveling to and from—and within—the United States shortly before she died of tuberculosis.[5] Most of the people she infected were seated near her in the back of the plane throughout the flight, but one was a flight attendant who was seated at the back of the plane only during takeoff and landing, and another was a passenger who apparently was infected while standing nearby in line for the toilets. During just 6 months in 1994, there were more than 30 other reports of passengers with active TB traveling on commercial flights in the United States.

As air travelers and airline crews know, the air on planes is not good. It flows into the cabin from overhead and out through vents near the floor. A lot of fuel is required to take in the thin, cold outside air at high altitudes, concentrate it, and warm it. Therefore, up to half of the cabin air is recirculated, and that increases the risk of infection, whether from your seatmate's cold or her tuberculosis. Usually the air is passed through filters. In the last few years, a number of airlines have installed high-efficiency particulate air (HEPA) filters that remove 99.7 percent of tiny particles the size of most bacteria from the recirculated air.[6] HEPA filters reduce the risk of infection, but they don't eliminate it. Furthermore, the ordinary passenger has no way of knowing whether a particular airplane has been equipped with HEPA filters.[7]

In 1996, after the incident with the Asian passenger, the CDC developed a protocol for public health authorities to follow in notifying passengers and crew who have been exposed to tuberculosis on an airplane. Like the World Health Organization, the CDC said that the risk was greatest for people on flights lasting 8 hours or more, for passengers and crew who were seated close to the index passenger, and in cases when the index passenger had advanced, very infectious TB.

Barry called the CDC Quarantine Station at JFK Airport in New York. He also called the airline, a major U.S. and international carrier. Airlines, as one might suspect, hate to get involved in this type of investigation, and their cooperation varies considerably. At first, the airline said the flight was under 8 hours—as if the danger developed only at *exactly* 8 hours. However, Nikolay had told investigators about the delay waiting for takeoff. That brought the time on the airplane to about 8 hours. In addition, there was the time taxiing to the gate in New York. Finally the airline conceded that the flight could be considered to have taken 8 hours, and the investigation could go ahead.

Now Barry's priority was to identify and notify the passengers who had been closest to the index case. How could the disease detectives find these passengers?

It took Bill Barry 3 months and much creative detective work to track down the passengers who had been sitting near Nikolay on the flight. From the airline's seating assignments, the CDC Quarantine Station at JFK found the names of the 36 people who were at highest risk of infection: those seated in the seven rows alongside, behind, and in front of the index case. If Barry and his colleagues found that tuberculosis had spread beyond those 36 nearest to Nikolay, they would extend the search to others on the airplane. Of course there was no way of knowing whether passengers had switched seats. Barry asked the airline to notify the crew members of their risk, but the airline never told him whether it had contacted the crew members, and it wouldn't allow him to contact the crew members directly.

Barry then went to work tracing these 36 passengers. He tracked them down through Form 990, the familiar customs declarations form that each passenger or family fills out, and which includes addresses; these forms are stored in a warehouse. Of the 36 passengers, three came from countries outside the United States and had given only hotel addresses, which they had long since left. There was no way to trace them to Argentina, Spain, or France. Were they businesspeople? Were they tourists? Did they bring their kids to see the White House or Disneyland? There was no way to know. "They fell through the cracks," Barry said.

The remaining 33 passengers came from New York City, New York State, California, Washington state, and Pennsylvania.

Two of them said that they had previously tested positive for tuberculosis infection on skin tests. Perhaps they had been infected as children but never developed the disease. They were given chest X-rays, which showed no signs of active tuberculosis. The other passengers included 17 from the Ukraine and 14 American-born individuals. Of this group, the Americans and 6 Ukranians had negative skin tests; 11 Ukrainians had positive ones. There was no way of knowing whether these were old infections, new infections caught from Nikolay, or a result of the (Bacille Calmette-Guérin [BCG] vaccine, a tuberculosis vaccine) vaccination given in childhood to most citizens of the former Soviet Union. There was no way to prove that these passengers had been recently infected by Nikolay on the airplane, and there was no way to prove that they hadn't been.

Given this information, the investigators gave a sigh of relief. There was no proof of transmission of TB from Nikolay to anyone who had traveled on the airplane. But still there were doubts. And what about other flights, probably hundreds of them, with an unknown, undiagnosed passenger with TB on board, a passenger who was never followed up in the careful way that

Nikolay was? No one notices when good public health procedures are followed—people notice only when they are not, and disaster happens.

Nikolay's wife had a positive skin test for tuberculosis, an indication that
she was infected with latent TB, but her chest X-ray did not show any sign
of active disease. Of Nikolay's seven relatives in the Pennsylvania community who had not been on the plane, five had negative skin tests; two had
positive ones. There was no way to know whether the two had new infections caught from Nikolay, old infections that their bodies had controlled,
or just positive skin tests because they had received the BCG vaccination
as children.

Meanwhile, Nikolay had active tuberculosis. But Barry and his colleagues
still didn't know whether this was ordinary tuberculosis, which could be
treated with the standard drug regimen, or multi-drug-resistant TB. The first
report on Nikolay's drug sensitivity tests came back in only a month, much
more quickly than usual. The Pennsylvania health department lab reported
that his tuberculosis was resistant to treatment with isoniazid, ethambutol,
and pyrazinamide—three of the five drugs used in first-line treatment of
tuberculosis. Worse yet, his strain of tuberculosis also seemed to be resistant
to three second-line drugs: kanamycin, ethionamide, and capreomycin,
which are used in cases of resistance to first-line drugs. The bottom line:
Nikolay and anyone unlucky enough to be infected by him had a strain of
tuberculosis that was resistant to an incredible six of the nine drugs used to
treat the disease.

Technically, Nikolay's tuberculosis was not multi-drug-resistant because
it was resistant only to isoniazid and not to rifampin. Luckily, rifampin could
still be used as part of his treatment. Still, it was unaffected by six of the
most powerful drugs used to treat tuberculosis.

Within a short time the other labs chimed in with their results. They
had similar findings for most of the drugs, but disagreed on some. That is
not unusual. Testing for resistance or sensitivity is a difficult, time-consuming
process, and there is room for discrepancy.

The good news was that all the labs agreed that Nikolay's tuberculosis
was sensitive to two powerful, first-line drugs: streptomycin and rifampin.

As soon as the Pennsylvania team got the results of the drug sensitivity
tests, they consulted with Dr. Patrick J. Brennan, an infectious diseases expert
at the University of Pennsylvania, who also directs the Philadelphia tuberculosis program. With the nod from Brennan, they put Nikolay's wife on a
course of rifampin, the drug they felt confident would kill off her latent
infection and prevent her from getting active tuberculosis. They switched
Nikolay to a strict regimen of drugs they believed his tuberculosis was

sensitive to: streptomycin, rifampin, ethionamide, and levofloxacin. Nevertheless, his sputum remained positive for tuberculosis bacteria when cultured six times, from September 5 through October 20, 1998. On November 24, 1998, for the first time, his sputum was negative when examined for acid-fast bacilli (TB bacteria) under the microscope. This was a good sign, although culture of his sputum still showed tuberculosis bacteria. On December 4, 1998, for the first time, both an acid-fast smear of his sputum and a culture of his sputum were negative. After that, until May 10, 1999, he had negative smears and cultures, excellent signs that the treatment was working. After May, he was unable to produce sputum—another sign that his tuberculosis was being treated successfully. He continued treatment for another 6 months after the last positive smear and culture. Sixteen months after he walked into the Erie County public health clinic, he was pronounced cured of drug-resistant tuberculosis. The cost of tracing and testing the people who were exposed to him on the airplane and in the community cannot be easily estimated. Whatever the cost, it was cheaper than dealing with an epidemic.

When people in Erie County heard about Nikolay, said Barry, "They were concerned about how he got into the country. I said, thank God he walked into the clinic in 3 days! He could have been in the community for 6 months, spreading tuberculosis that was resistant to six drugs." Barry feels that the Pennsylvania town was very, very lucky.

Of course no one can know whether Nikolay, the index case, spread tuberculosis to other people whom he came in contact with on his journey from the former Soviet Union to Erie County, Pennsylvania. Only if they get sick will they know that they've been infected. And then some doctor somewhere, knowing nothing of his or her patient's history, will begin the arduous task of figuring out what the patient has and ultimately, if and when TB is diagnosed, what drugs can cure this particular strain of resistant tuberculosis.

2

Cows and Mummies: A Brief History of Tuberculosis

Tuberculosis originally spread from animals to humans, just as AIDS did in the twentieth century. It probably leaped from cows to humans about 8,000 or 10,000 years ago, when people first settled down in communities to tend their cattle and plant their crops. Farmers and herders lived in close quarters with their animals. Perhaps they even welcomed the warmth from cows living in stalls beneath or alongside their family quarters. They still live this way in primitive and isolated areas.

From their cows, some farmers and their families probably contracted an airborne infection called *Mycobacterium bovis*. Sick cows exhaled the bacteria, and human beings breathed them in. They may also have gotten TB bacteria from the cows' milk. The bacteria learned to live in the human body, which is not all that different from a cow's, preferring to settle in the lungs, although they could attack many other organs. Over the years, the bacteria from the cows probably mutated slightly into *M. tuberculosis*. Indeed, *M. bovis* and *M. tuberculosis* are astonishingly alike—so similar that they and two other related bugs are grouped together as the *M. tuberculosis* complex.[1]

Mycobacterium tuberculosis grew and thrived in human bodies and spread from one sick man or woman to another. Wherever people settled, TB came with them. Characteristic scars of tuberculosis have been found in the bones of ancient Egyptian mummies. In 460 B.C., the Greek physician Hippocrates described tuberculosis as an "almost always fatal disease of the lungs."[2] The Greeks called the disease phthisis (pronounced "TEE-sis"), which may be derived from the Greek word for wasting or decay.[3] (To this day, specialists in tuberculosis are called phthisiologists.) Today *M. tuberculosis* infects 2 billion people—one-third of the world's population. Every year more than 8 million people progress to active, usually infectious, TB, and this number is growing. A person with active TB typically infects another 20 people: This means 160 million new infections every year. Each and every year, 2 to 3 million people will die from the disease.

In the Air

In one way, TB is dangerously *unlike* HIV, the virus that causes AIDS. That virus can be spread only by intimate sexual contact, exchanges of blood, or from mother to child through childbirth or from breastfeeding. Tuberculosis is far more promiscuous. It flies through the air whenever the afflicted person coughs or sneezes or sings or laughs or, sometimes, just talks. With each cough, a spray of moisture erupts from a person's nose or mouth. If the person has active TB, the spray may include millions of droplets loaded with TB bacteria as their nuclei. The moisture in the droplets dries up quickly, but the droplet nuclei can hang in the air for hours, particularly in dark, cramped quarters where the ultraviolet rays of sunlight cannot reach them to kill them. These lethal nuclei can infect anyone who breathes them in.

Air is breathed in through the nose or mouth, and goes down through the trachea, or windpipe, and then into two tubes called mainstem bronchi, one to each lung. From there it passes into the lobes of the lungs. The right lung has three lobes; the left lung has two. Each lobe is like a cluster of grapes or a sponge, full of small air spaces called alveoli. This is where the important business of breathing goes on. Blood vessels lie just below the surface membrane of each alveolus. The blood vessels send the body's waste product of respiration, carbon dioxide, out into the alveoli, where it will be expelled with the next breath. In exchange, they pick up oxygen from the incoming air and send it to the tissues throughout the body, including the brain and muscles. If the lungs stop working, the brain will die from lack of oxygen in about 4 minutes, and the entire body will die soon after.

Human bodies normally have excellent defenses, so it's not easy for TB-carrying droplets or droplet nuclei to travel deep down into the lungs, where they must lodge in order to cause infection. Many droplets are caught on the tiny, hairlike cells that line the body's airways. They then may be swept up and expelled through the nose, or be swept into the throat, swallowed, and destroyed by the stomach acids. The smaller the droplets are, the more likely they are to be inhaled deep down into the air spaces of the lungs.

Suppose a tiny droplet containing TB bacteria does make it deep into a person's lungs and lodges within one of those small alveoli with a rich blood supply. What happens? The outcome depends on several things: How big was the dose of TB bacteria? How strong is the person's immune system to fight off the infection? How virulent, malignant, and dangerous are the TB germs that were inhaled?

No one knows how many bacteria are usually needed to start a human tuberculosis infection. We know that it is possible for a single droplet nucleus of TB bacteria to do the trick,[4] but we also know from experience that infection is far more likely after lengthy exposure. Occasionally a person will catch TB after a brief encounter in a bus or on a subway, in an airplane, or in an emergency room, but someone else may not be infected even when a close family member has active TB for months. Spending hours at home, at work, or in school with somebody who has untreated, active TB day after day for weeks and months makes it far more likely that a healthy person will become infected, but even then, infection might not occur. We think that genetic differences between human beings may play a role in determining who will become infected after exposure to TB bacteria, and we think that the virulence of the particular strain of TB bacteria may be a factor, but we don't really know. Even though we have been at the mercy of this ravaging and enigmatic disease for 10,000 years, there is little hard knowledge and much speculation about how it picks its victims. Sometimes it's just a matter of luck.

Suppose a person is unlucky. What happens when the droplet with active TB bacteria finds a small, warm home deep in one of the alveoli of the lung? First, the body's advance defense cells, called macrophages, rush to the area of infection and try to swallow up the invading bacteria. But TB bacteria are tough nuts to crack. They have hard, waxy coats that are difficult to penetrate. Bacteria are most vulnerable when they are in the act of multiplying, but *M. tuberculosis* multiplies very slowly—only once in 20–24 hours, whereas most common bacteria multiply as often as every 20 minutes. This doesn't give the macrophages many opportunities to attack. So the macrophages encircle the TB bacteria and enclose them in a sort of membrane. We have seen this in animal studies, and we think the same thing happens in humans, but we don't know for sure whether macrophages can kill TB bacteria in humans in this way or can only contain them and stop them from multiplying. We assume that sometimes the TB bacteria are not killed, because people with a latent TB infection (as shown by a positive tuberculin skin test) may develop active tuberculosis when they grow older or when their immune systems are weakened by another disease.

We do know that if the macrophages succeed in killing or immobilizing the TB bacteria, the infection is stopped right there. But if the TB bacteria win this initial skirmish and kill the macrophages, then tuberculosis infection begins in earnest. More macrophages rush in to stem the invasion.

The TB bacteria, like the opportunistic parasites they are, break into the macrophages and begin multiplying inside them. Then they burst out through the walls of the helpless and spent defense cells. Desperately, other macrophages rush in and gobble up the debris, only to be commandeered by the TB bacteria. The bacteria stick together in an ever-growing cluster. The macrophages can't penetrate to the center of this growing clump of infection.

The TB bacteria continue this cycle of devouring macrophages and growing for several weeks, creating a microscopic, tumorlike nodule. This dangerous lump is called a tubercle, from which the disease derives its name. The tubercle sends out daughter cells through the bloodstream and through the lymph that drain the lungs. Thus the TB infection spreads, actually metastasizing somewhat like cancer.

After about 3 or 4 weeks of struggling, the body's immune defenses usually gain the upper hand over the TB bacteria. Although the bacteria are not killed, they are walled off into lumps of scar tissue, the tubercles. The majority of the TB bacteria remain latent within the tubercles, waiting. The mixture of dead bacteria, latent bacteria, and macrophages that fills the tubercles looks like cheese, and is often described as "caseous," meaning "cheeselike." In most people the infection stays latent, confined within the tubercle, for the rest of their lives. A chest X-ray of these people may show very small areas of scar tissue in their lungs. If they have a tuberculin skin test, it will be positive. Both are signs of infection, whether the infection occurred in the distant past or much more recently. Treatment of the latent infection at this point is highly effective in preventing future active tuberculosis.

Some people are unlucky. In about 1 in 10 cases, the initial infection is never completely controlled by the body's defenses. In about half of this unlucky 10 percent, the infection progresses immediately or within the first few years to active, often infectious, tuberculosis, a debilitating, wasting disease. In the other half, it does so after a delay of up to several decades. In active tuberculosis, whether in the first few years after infection or much later, as the tuberculosis bacteria multiply, they eat away and destroy the healthy lung tissue, creating ulcerlike cavities full of highly infectious pus and tuberculosis bacteria in the spongelike structure of the lungs. These pockets of disease replace normal, healthy lung tissue and may impair the victim's ability to breathe. Unlike skin, which grows back after cuts and scratches, damaged lung tissue usually does not repair itself without scarring. Increasingly, the patient coughs because of irritation of the lining of the lung or to expel the phlegm and pus that fills the cavities. A lung cavity

1 inch in diameter may contain 100 million TB bacteria. As the person coughs, sneezes, sings, or laughs, infectious TB bacteria may spew out into the air.

Sometimes the bacteria spread to the bones, causing abscesses and deformities of the shoulders, hips, legs, or spine. A typical TB bony deformity of the upper spine may cause a hunchback, a condition we now call Pott's disease. (This is probably what afflicted the Hunchback of Notre Dame.) Sometimes the bacteria move on to destroy the kidneys or move to the gastrointestinal tract, where they may cause frequent, unpredictable, devastating diarrhea.

TB bacteria may also infect lymph nodes, especially the ones at the side of the neck below the ears. Here they can eat through to the skin, causing draining sores called scrofula. These sores were known as "the king's evil" in England and France, where the touch of a king or queen was thought to cure them. Samuel Johnson, who compiled the first English dictionary, was "touched for the evil" by Queen Anne on March 30, 1712, at the age of 2¹/₂.[5] Queen Anne, who died in 1714, was the last sovereign of Great Britain to touch for the evil.[6]

An International Disease

Over the centuries, tuberculosis became a common, often epidemic disease.

Tuberculosis kept steadily killing throughout Egyptian, Greek, Roman, medieval, and Renaissance times, although overshadowed by more sudden and spectacular outbreaks of plague, smallpox, dysentery, leprosy, syphilis, and other ills. Since tuberculosis spreads most easily when people are in close contact with an infected person who is coughing or sneezing, it was probably more common in towns than among the peasants in the countryside.[7] People came to towns to trade their goods, sell their produce, or carry on other business. They met in taverns and lived in cramped quarters at the inns, with several people to a room. If they moved to town to make their fortune or to escape the yoke of serfdom, they often found cheap accommodations where they shared not only cramped rooms but even beds. In the sixteenth through the nineteenth centuries, many of the new arrivals in the major cities of Europe were consumed by tuberculosis or other infectious diseases.[8] A city's population was maintained only by a steady supply of healthy young people coming to make their fortunes.

Still, city dwellers were relatively few. Most people lived in the countryside as peasants and farmers, and they spent much of their time out of doors. If they were ill, they coughed tuberculosis bacteria into the open air, where the ultraviolet rays in the sunlight killed them. (Ultraviolet lights are used today in hospitals, homeless shelters, and laboratories to kill tuberculosis bacteria in the air.) Even if peasants infected their families in their small huts, country life was isolated, and it was unlikely that tuberculosis would spread from village to village. The infected people were far away from the larger society to which they could spread their infection.

The Industrial Revolution, which began in the late seventeenth century in England and perhaps a hundred years later in the United States, brought more people into the urban centers, and city life became more perilous. Men, women, and children were packed cheek-by-jowl into huge, poorly ventilated industrial factories (the poet William Blake called them "dark satanic mills").

Even in their own homes, away from the factories, people could not escape the stagnant air in which disease can flourish. In 1696, the British government began to tax windows to make up for the revenue that it lost when people trimmed off the edges of gold and silver coins.[9] Naturally, people began stopping up windows to avoid taxation. Notorious as the "tax on light and air," the law was not repealed until 1851. A similar window tax existed in France.

It thus became a luxury to have light, air, and breezes in your home or lodging. Sunlight kills TB bacteria, and air exchange through breezes sweeps TB bacteria away and dilutes their concentration, but a property owner could save money by bricking up windows and still renting the crowded, damp, dark quarters to families who lived several to a room. In 1901, 36 percent of Dublin's housing units consisted of a single room. Almost every one of those single rooms—98 percent—had at least five occupants.[10] Alcoholism and poor nutrition made the situation even more dire, degrading immune systems and making people more susceptible to tuberculosis.

In the eastern United States, young women moved from farms across New England to textile centers like Lowell, to work in the mills and to taste a more exciting life than the farm could offer. Young men moved to the city, working at any job they could find. This was a time of enormous immigration from Ireland, Germany, and, later, southern Europe to the United States. Tuberculosis killed many of those bright young people who came to town to make their fortune and the immigrants who hoped they could lead a better, safer life than at home.

Not only were people in Europe and the United States crowded into single rooms, but they were also sardined into prison cells. According to Thomas Dormandy, "between 1870 and 1880 half of all prisoners in Chatham Naval Prison [near London] developed galloping tuberculosis every winter and died. No lifer in an American prison survived more than 12 years before 1910 and between 1890 and 1895. Tuberculosis was the listed cause of death in three-quarters of the prison population in Massachusetts."[11]

All of these factors together created the perfect breeding ground for TB, which became epidemic in the seventeenth, eighteenth, and nineteenth centuries in Europe, and in the nineteenth century in the United States.[12] In the seventeenth century, case rates, or the number of new cases per 100,000 people per year, were astonishingly high, probably reaching 1000 or 1250 in London.[13] One-quarter of the population of Europe probably suffered from tuberculosis at that time.[14] In the early eighteenth century, TB caused about one-third of all deaths in Europe.[15] According to Sheila Rothman, during this period tuberculosis caused one-fifth of all deaths in the United States,[16] and it remained a leading cause of death in the United States well into the twentieth century.[17]

Whether rich or poor, merchant or servant, the victim of tuberculosis often became thin, pale, and exhausted. He or she began to cough, and then to cough more often, trying to remove the lethal and irritating bacteria-clogged pus from lungs and airways. As the disease progressed, the victim coughed up floods of sputum and phlegm and suffered agonizing pains in the chest. The sputum became stained with blood. The victim often wasted away, becoming a thing of skin and bones with eyes sunk deep in a skeletal face. It seemed as if the body was being consumed from within, and so the disease came to be called consumption. Sometimes death arrived relatively peacefully and the victim quietly faded away. Other times he or she would actually drown from a sudden hemorrhage when the tuberculosis cavities in the lungs ate into blood vessels, which burst, so that blood flooded into the corroded lungs and poured from the nose and mouth. Before effective antibiotics became available, probably half of TB patients died within 5 years—a far, far worse death rate than that for most cancers today—and some died within a few weeks of raging disease, called "galloping consumption." The others lived longer, usually sickly lives, frequently interrupted by unpredictable relapses of their disease. Throughout their illness, they often spread the disease to those around them.

For thousands of years, no one knew that tuberculosis was an infectious disease. In the nineteenth century, doctors in western Europe and the United States were sure that tuberculosis was hereditary because it so often ran in families. In fact, it ran in families because families lived in the same house—sometimes in the same room—and infected each other through their shared air.

Many tuberculosis sufferers in Europe and the United States traveled to milder climates, which were thought to be beneficial for patients with this disease. George Washington sailed to Barbados in the West Indies with his half-brother Lawrence in 1751 in an attempt to cure Lawrence's tuberculosis.[18] But Lawrence died in Barbados. George Washington himself suffered several illnesses that might have been tuberculosis; he himself called them consumption.[19]

A Romantic Disease

Perhaps because in the nineteenth century so many of the best, brightest, most glamorous young people died from tuberculosis, it became a romantic disease. Like AIDS today, it seemed to single out the young and talented —writers, poets, and playwrights; artists; musicians; courtesans; scientists; and society beauties. People dying of tuberculosis became thin, pale, and gaunt, a look that was considered stylish, much like today's "heroin chic" supermodels. They were the subjects of countless paintings, poems, and operas. Think of Camille, the Lady of the Camellias, pining away; of Mimi dying of TB in a Parisian slum in *La Bohème;* or of Violetta singing her last aria in *La Traviata*. Victims of consumption were feverish and, as the disease progressed, exhausted. But they were also thought to have a special hot-headed impetus that drove them to frantic sexual activity and great creativity in the arts.

Most of us have read about the Romantic poet John Keats. As a teenager, he devoted himself to caring for his mother while she was dying of tuberculosis. He remained apparently healthy, trained as a doctor, and passed his exams in 1816, at the age of 20. Nevertheless, he decided to dedicate himself to poetry. He led a vigorous life, with long hikes through some of England's most beautiful countryside. However, he almost certainly had caught tuberculosis from his mother or from his brother Tom, whom he also spent nearly a year taking care of, sleeping in the same room with him. Tom died of tuberculosis in 1818.

On a cold night in London, on February 3, 1820, John Keats coughed up blood on his pillow. As a doctor, he knew what it meant. He said to the friend he was staying with, "I know the colour of that blood—it is arterial blood—I cannot be deceived in that colour; that drop of blood is my death warrant. I must die."[20] Keats traveled to the milder climate of Italy in hopes of a recovery, but he died in Rome a year later, on February 23, 1821.[21]

The members of the talented Brontë family fell like dominoes to TB. The Brontës lived in a grim, cold parsonage in Haworth in Yorkshire,

England, in the early nineteenth century, and the girls were sent to a strict boarding school, where they lived in cold, crowded dormitory rooms and received skimpy meals. Patrick Brontë, a Methodist minister, his wife, Maria, and their six children all developed TB. Patrick may have been the source, or the girls may have picked it up at school and spread it to their family when they came home. Maria, the mother, may have died of a childbirth infection, or she may have died of tuberculosis. The daughter Maria was ill and came home to die at the age of 12. Elizabeth died a month later at age 11. The others lived to grow up, but they did not escape tuberculosis. Branwell, the only boy in the family, died in 1848. Emily, who wrote *Wuthering Heights*, died a month later, and Anne died 6 months after Emily, at age 29. Charlotte, who wrote *Jane Eyre*, died at 38, in a pregnancy complicated by tuberculosis. Of the entire Brontë family, only Patrick survived to old age.[22]

The list of famous people who died from tuberculosis is long. René Laennec, a French physician, invented the stethoscope around 1818 or 1819 so that he could better hear the sounds within patients' chests. It was the best tool for diagnosing tuberculosis that doctors had until the end of the nineteenth century. Laennec himself died of tuberculosis in 1826, when he was only 45.[23] Thomas Wakley (1795-1862), the doctor who founded the internationally known medical journal *Lancet*, died of tuberculosis while on a rest cure on the island of Madeira, known for its mild climate.[24]

Henry David Thoreau and the composer Frédéric Chopin both died of tuberculosis in the 1800s. Fyodor Dostoyevsky, the Russian novelist, wrote of tuberculosis in *The House of the Dead* and died from the disease in 1881. A TB hospital in Moscow is named for him.

Tuberculosis continued killing the brilliant and the ordinary well into the twentieth century; among those who died were the Russian doctor and playwright Anton Chekhov and Edward Livingston Trudeau, the father of the TB sanatorium movement in the United States, who died of tuberculosis in 1915. The Italian artist Amadeo Modigliani and the Czech writer Franz Kafka also succumbed to TB, as did Katherine Mansfield and George Orwell.

First Lady Eleanor Roosevelt died of tuberculosis in 1962 at Columbia-Presbyterian Medical Center, a major teaching hospital in New York City. The story goes that her doctors had not recognized the disease and had treated it incorrectly, using steroids that suppressed her immune system and made it easier for the tuberculosis to flourish.[25] However, recently Dr. Barron Lerner of Columbia-Presbyterian found the original notes from the case and learned that Roosevelt had been properly treated with the TB drugs available at that time, isoniazid and streptomycin. Her doctors thought she was suffering a recurrence of TB that she had caught as a young woman. But the drugs did not work, and Roosevelt died. Only after her death did the Columbia lab get the results of drug-sensitivity testing and find that, to their surprise, Roosevelt's TB was resistant to both isoniazid and streptomycin. Thus, her disease could not have been a recurrence of an early infection, because the drugs had not yet been discovered when she was young; she died of TB that she had recently caught. Isoniazid and streptomycin had been in use for only 15 years or less, and already there were resistant strains of TB bacteria.[26]

Magic Mountains

Over all these centuries, no one knew what caused this devastating disease. However, the clammy, cold, damp climate of northern Europe and the northern United States was thought to make it worse. Many of those who could afford it sought out a milder climate or clear mountain air. Switzerland became a health destination, and towns like Davos were full of sanatoriums, which combined the features of a hospital with those of a luxury hotel. Sanatoriums offered a regimen like those of today's spas: a healthy environment, good nutrition, and gradually increasing exercise. The lifestyle change forced upon TB sufferers was considerable. The highly regimented stay in a sanatorium ranged from 2 to sometimes as much as 5 or even 10 years, and was romanticized in novels like Thomas Mann's *The Magic Mountain*, published in 1927. When TB declined in the twentieth century, the sanatoriums often became hotels catering to skiers, hikers, tourists, and celebrities.

In the United States, the sanatorium movement was started by Dr. Edward L. Trudeau, who had become dangerously ill with tuberculosis. In 1873, he moved to the Adirondack Mountains in northern New York State, not because he thought it would improve his health, but because he planned to end his days among the lakes and mountains that he loved.[27] Dr. Trudeau found that fresh air and rest, particularly outdoors, had a restorative effect on his spirits and his health, and so, with help from friends, he established a sanatorium near Saranac Lake.

For a while the mountain air improved Dr. Trudeau's health, but repetitive bouts of active tuberculosis continued to destroy his lungs. During the course of the next 42 years, he was often ill, but he continued his research in tuberculosis. He helped found the National Association for the Study and Prevention of Tuberculosis, now the American Lung Association, still the most important voluntary organization dealing with tuberculosis, and in

1904 served as its first president.[28] He finally succumbed to his illness in 1915, despite having undergone what was then the latest therapy: collapsing a lung through a method called pneumothorax.

Trudeau's sanatorium movement flourished in the United States, probably to excess. By 1923, there were 656 sanatoriums with 66,000 beds.[29] People who were unable to leave home and go to a sanatorium would seek out fresh air by sleeping in a tent on the roof of their tenement or on the porch of their house, or by attending school in the open air. Hospitals built in that era usually have extended porch areas, which were originally intended to allow TB patients to benefit from fresh air.

The sanatorium movement, with its draconian demands on a patient's life, seems archaic today, and sanatoriums had absolutely no effect in curing TB. The death rate was about the same. Whether tuberculosis patients were treated in a sanatorium or not treated at all, half of them died. But sanatoriums did accomplish two things: (1) They removed people with active, infectious tuberculosis from their communities. Once in a sanatorium, an infectious person could no longer spread his or her disease to family, friends, coworkers, employers, or other people around him or her. (2) The entire specialty of pulmonary medicine took root. The physicians at these sanatoriums, many patients themselves, later became interested as well in other aspects of lung disease such as asthma, emphysema, and lung cancer.

3

The World Is Different Now

The world changed on the evening of March 24, 1882, when a thin, near-sighted, 38-year-old German physician, Robert Koch, read a paper to the Physiological Society in Berlin.[1] Koch had already made a name for himself by identifying the cause of anthrax, a disease that was killing German cattle. He had also developed a way to dry and stain bacteria for examination under the microscope and a way to grow bacteria in culture, techniques that are still used all over the world today.

On that March evening in Berlin, Koch noted that "one-seventh of all human beings die of tuberculosis and . . . if one considers only the productive middle-age groups, tuberculosis carries away one-third and often more of these."[2] Reading his brilliant paper through his thick glasses, Koch told his audience that tuberculosis *was an infectious disease caused by a bacterium*. He spelled out the scientific evidence to prove this in meticulous detail. It was astonishing news. At last, the cause of the disease that had terrified humanity possibly more than any other disease for millennia had been identified. When Koch finished his presentation, the audience sat in stunned silence.

Koch's news was just as shattering to his listeners as the news that the earth was round, not flat, had been to their ancestors. This was a profound change, a revolution in scientific thinking. The doctors and scientists in that Berlin hall had just heard that the major killer disease of their time was not inherited and was not mysterious. It was an infectious disease that was spread through the air by bacteria. That meant that one day it might be prevented and cured.

A well-known physician, Paul Ehrlich, who discovered the "magic bullet" (salvarsan) for syphilis and won the Nobel Prize, was in the audience. He later wrote, "In simple terms, understandable by all, Koch explained the etiology of tuberculosis and provided convincing evidence. All those present

23

were greatly struck and I must admit that this evening stands in my memory as my greatest scientific experience."[3] Koch, too, won the Nobel Prize
for medicine and physiology, the world's highest recognition in this field, in
1905. Since the centennial of Koch's momentous discovery, and following
a proposal from Mali in 1991, the International Union Against Tuberculosis
and Lung Disease, the World Health Organization, the U.S. Centers for
Disease Control and Prevention, the American Lung Association, and cru-
saders against tuberculosis celebrate March 24 as World TB Day. In 2002,
the 120th anniversary of Koch's discovery, more than 200 countries and nongovernmental organizations will simultaneously conduct public outreach
activities.

Through an elegant four-step procedure that scientists still use and refer
to as "Koch's postulates," Koch methodically showed that the tuberculosis
bacteria did indeed cause the disease.[4] First, he isolated tuberculosis bacteria from animals with "consumption." Second, he grew the bacteria in culture. Third, he inoculated healthy animals with the bacteria and waited. The
healthy animals became ill with the symptoms of "consumption" and died.
Fourth, he recovered tuberculosis bacteria from the animals that died.
Although tuberculosis could affect almost any organ of the body, Koch
learned that it usually made its entry through the lungs, when someone
inhaled droplets that had been coughed out by a person with the disease.

At first, the shocked scientific establishment, in Germany and elsewhere,
refused to believe that bacteria caused tuberculosis. How could well-
meaning, good, dedicated physicians have been wrong for so many years?
How could tiny, invisible bacteria cause this devastating disease that killed
so many? Was it at all possible that tuberculosis was *not* inherited? The controversy went on for years and became part of a larger international debate
over the germ theory itself. Many scientists found it difficult to believe that
germs could cause *any* disease at all. Some dug in their heels and refused to
consider the evidence that Koch had so carefully amassed, stubbornly
believing until they went to their graves that TB was hereditary.

Despite the controversy, however, it quickly became apparent that
Koch's discovery had opened up a whole new world. Soon, doctors would
benefit from a much more scientific approach to their old foe. To begin with,
the disease was now called tuberculosis, instead of the vague "consumption."
Doctors no longer had to rely on the nonspecific symptoms of cough, weight
loss, fevers, and night sweats to make the diagnosis. They could examine the
patient's sputum under the microscope and look for the telltale tuberculosis bacteria. For the first time, the presence of the tiny rods could distinguish
tuberculosis from other lung problems and infections.

Thirteen years after Koch identified the cause of tuberculosis, William Konrad Roentgen discovered X-rays (also called Roentgen rays) while studying electrical discharge in a high-vacuum tube. With X-rays, doctors could see into the body and view the scar tissue or inflammation caused by tuberculosis in the lungs. Air and healthy air-containing tissue (like the spongy lungs) appear black on a lung X-ray. Inflammation in lung tissue, fluid, or pus show up clearly in white. Doctors could relate a patient's signs and symptoms to the damage they saw on the X-ray plate. Originally, each image was stored on a fragile 14- × 17-inch piece of glass. X-rays quickly became an essential tool in medicine, and Roentgen received the first Nobel Prize in physics.

Having identified the enemy under the microscope and seen in X-rays the scars and cavities caused by TB, scientists could begin to search for a cure and develop ways to protect the public from this deadly infectious disease. Koch's seminal discovery led scientists and health officials to realize that people with active tuberculosis could be a serious danger to everyone around them. Tuberculosis was more common among the poor and immigrants, but it was clear that it was spread through the air. Everyone had to breathe, so even then as now, social class was no protection. Obviously, even the wealthy were exposed, because they employed the poor as servants or came into contact with them in public places.

Public health officials, assisted by voluntary nongovernmental organizations such as the National Association for the Study and Prevention of Tuberculosis (predecessor of the American Lung Association), began campaigns to reduce the spread of tuberculosis.[5] Spitting was prohibited, because infected sputum spat out by someone with active TB was thought to be a major cause of infection. (It isn't. The key to infection is that TB bacteria spread as an aerosol, tiny, moist particles that may hang in the air for hours or be carried by a ventilation system to a different room, as happened in an outbreak on the U.S. Navy destroyer U.S.S. *Byrd* in 1965.[6] A blob of spit [or sputum] usually settles quickly on the floor and doesn't become an aerosol. It certainly isn't pleasant, but it's not a way of spreading TB.) In 1887, the first TB control system was established in Edinburgh, Scotland, by Sir Robert W. Phillip.[7] His ambitious program included public education, aggressive diagnosis, mandatory reporting of patients to public health authorities, record keeping, examination of sputum for TB bacteria, social services, a dispensary, home visits by doctors and nurses, and follow-up care. It served as a model for many other cities, and all of these elements are applicable today.

In New York City, a report in 1893 by Dr. Hermann Biggs, who later became the city's pioneering health commissioner, recommended a public education campaign, disinfection of the homes or hospital rooms of TB patients, separation of TB patients from other patients in hospitals, the establishment of a special hospital for TB patients, and diagnostic examination of sputum in patients with pulmonary disease, at the doctor's request.[8] In an effort to protect close contacts from infection, he also advocated requiring doctors to notify the health department of all TB cases within 7 days of diagnosis. Doctors in New York and elsewhere objected to compulsory notification, but the rule took hold. Today tuberculosis is still one of the few "notifiable diseases"—diseases that doctors must report to public health authorities for the protection of the community. Compulsory notification remains an important public health tool.

Just the Facts

By the beginning of the twentieth century, both doctors and the public had grasped the basic facts about tuberculosis: (1) It was caused by bacteria. (2) It most often infected the lungs. (3) It spread through the air when an infected person coughed, sneezed, laughed, spoke, or sang. And (4), its spread could be halted by isolating the infected person from the community. Diagnosis became more accurate as a result of Koch's discovery of the TB bacteria, which led to the test we still use today, more than a century later: the acid-fast smear. In this process, doctors stain a sample of sputum with chemicals and look for the characteristic TB bacteria.[9] For final, certain diagnosis, scientists could put the sputum in a culture dish and, using proper temperature and nutrients, encourage any tuberculosis bacteria to grow. However, these bacteria grow very slowly. Specific growth and biochemical characteristics for TB could be observed, confirming the diagnosis. It might be a month or more before doctors could absolutely identify TB bacteria in the culture. This technique, which is also more than a century old, is still the gold standard for diagnosis of TB. Unfortunately, until the early 1950s, even though they could now make an accurate diagnosis, there still wasn't much doctors could do for a patient with signs of tuberculosis as there were no drugs. Doctors could diagnose TB with bone-chilling accuracy, but they still could not treat it. Worse yet, the randomized controlled clinical trial to prove the efficacy of one treatment compared to another had not yet been invented. It was first adopted in the late 1940s; prior to then, assumptions of efficacy of treatments that might appear ludicrous today were often accepted—erroneously.

Doctors made a number of attempts at interventions, including some drastic surgical approaches that were probably worse than the disease. One of their ideas was complete resting of the diseased lung. Doctors had noticed that bed rest seemed to help TB patients, and by extension it was proposed that resting a diseased lung might help heal the TB cavities inside it. The whole idea of rest—for the lung and for the patient—was wrong. Patients were told to rest, and many of them survived, so it appeared that the bed rest was helping or even curing their TB. But it might have been just luck or a good immune system that brought about their cure—not the bed rest. No one made a systematic comparison of the outcomes in patients who were treated with bed rest and those who were not.

The idea of resting the lung started in 1696 when a Roman physician, Giorgio Baglivi, reported that a patient with tuberculosis had improved dramatically after he suffered a sword wound to his chest.[10] When the sword pierced the man's chest, air rushed in through the wound and filled the space between the lung and the chest wall. The air pressed against the lung and collapsed it. This accidental discovery prompted surgeons to try to repeat the process intentionally in a treatment called pneumothorax, meaning air in the chest (but outside the lung itself).

Pneumothorax could be used only on one side of the chest at one time. If both lungs were collapsed, the patient would be unable to breathe and would die within minutes. Thus, the procedure was suitable only for patients whose tuberculosis was confined to one lung, which could be determined by X-rays. Furthermore, pneumothorax could not be used in patients whose damaged lungs had become attached to the chest wall. Normally the lungs float inside the chest, but sometimes disease breaks through from the lung to the space between it and the chest wall, adhering the lung to the chest wall with scar tissue. When that occurs, there is no way to collapse the lung.

In the 1920s and 1930s, doctors would inject air or other gases into the chest cavity to collapse the lung. They had to repeat the procedure many times, as the air would soon be absorbed by the body, and the lung would reexpand. During this period, it was common for patients to go to an outpatient clinic for "pneumothorax refills," which were performed with a machine that allowed a precise amount of air to be injected into the chest. Since a pneumothorax of necessity could only be done by a physician, this was the earliest example of directly observed therapy.

Sometimes ribs on one side of the body were removed in an operation called a thoracoplasty to make the chest fall in and permanently collapse the lung. This was a brutal and disfiguring operation. Advocates of the operation claimed that the disfigurement was not noticeable under clothing. Other commonly used methods of collapsing the lung were cutting a nerve or injecting air into the abdomen to push the diaphragm up. Sometimes Lucite balls like Ping-Pong balls or thick, heavy oil were inserted into the chest to keep the lung collapsed, but such draconian surgical procedures often led to major complications like infection, embolism, and death. No comparison of pneumothorax or these other treatments was ever done. If pneumothorax helped any patients at all, it was probably because the collapse sealed off the diseased lung and prevented TB from spreading. Nonetheless, even though the science that went into these heavy-handed measures was lacking and there were no controlled trials, as would be required under current standards, Dr. Michael Iseman and his group at National Jewish Center in Denver have reported reasonable results at the present time using these otherwise obsolete methods in patients who are resistant to antituberculosis drugs, and therefore have no other treatment options.

On occasion doctors used surgery to remove a piece of a diseased lung or even the whole lung, thinking that the operation would eliminate the core of the infection and give the patient's body a better chance to fight off the disease. Improvements in anesthesia and in infection control during the nineteenth century made it possible to attempt such an operation. According to Dr. Ann Davis, a TB expert and historian, the first patient, operated on in 1883,[11] died. It wasn't until 1934 that surgeons performed the first successful removal of a lobe and then a whole lung for the treatment of TB. Even as late as 1943, 20 to 40 percent of these surgically treated patients died. Today, since antibiotic treatment to cure TB is widely available, surgery is usually considered a last, desperate measure for treating those cases of TB that are resistant to most or all drugs. For such patients, removing the core of the infection may help by diminishing the number of TB bacteria that must be fought by their immune systems and by their doctors' best remaining drugs. With fewer bacteria to fight, the patient (and the drugs) sometimes may have a better chance. And if the TB is localized in one lung, it can sometimes be eliminated altogether by surgery.

Only in the former Soviet Union is surgery for TB still considered a standard treatment, performed on thousands of patients each year. Almost every one of these patients could be cured by an outpatient regimen of cheap and effective drugs.

Removing a lung or part of a lung is a brutal procedure. At Newark's University Hospital, the hospital used by the New Jersey Medical School National Tuberculosis Center, we usually do no more than five of these operations a year, invariably on people who have neglected their TB for years and dropped out of good outpatient treatment programs. Their lungs have become a huge festering source of drug-resistant tuberculosis, and surgery is our last resort.

Promise of a Vaccine

Many diseases can be prevented today by immunization. In the past, folk wisdom said that there were some diseases you couldn't get twice: smallpox, for example. If a person survived an attack of smallpox, he or she would never get it again. The reason, we now know, is that the first attack primes the body's immune system. If the immune system sees the same invading bug again, it is prepared to destroy it.

In 1798, Edward Jenner, an English country doctor, discovered that infection with a mild disease, cowpox, could prevent infection with the related but much more serious smallpox. Jenner observed that milkmaids, who frequently caught cowpox from their cows, were immune to the dreaded smallpox. He hypothesized that deliberately introducing cowpox bacteria into the skin of an uninfected person might protect the individual from smallpox. In an audacious experiment that could never be conducted today for ethical reasons, he tried the technique on a healthy 8-year-old boy, inoculating him with cowpox bacteria and later challenging his immune system by injecting him with virulent smallpox bacteria. The child did not become ill: His system, primed by the cowpox vaccination,[12] protected him against the smallpox.

A good vaccine, like the smallpox vaccine, can produce miracles. Through an intensive worldwide vaccination effort, smallpox was eliminated from the planet in 1979.

Robert Koch knew about vaccination when he was working on tuberculosis in the last decades of the nineteenth century. His eminent contemporary Louis Pasteur had developed a vaccine against rabies, a disease that is still always fatal if it is not treated by immediate vaccination.[13] Pasteur took infected spinal cord tissue from rabid dogs ("mad dogs" that could infect anyone they attacked) and injected the tissue into rabbits. When the rabbits became ill, he took infected material from them and injected it into other rabbits. He repeated the process many times to weaken the virus. Then he injected the tissue into dogs to see if the dogs became rabid. They did not. In July 1885, a family brought him a young boy, Joseph Meisner, who 2 days previously had been badly bitten by a rabid dog. Pasteur's vaccine was the child's only hope. After consulting with colleagues, who agreed with him, he injected the boy with the weakened virus from the rabbits and gave him 12 more painful injections over the next 10 days. Joseph lived.

The technique Pasteur developed is called attenuating, or weakening, a virus. It is used today to produce vaccines such as the Sabin vaccine against polio. Such vaccines are also called "live virus" vaccines because the virus, although weakened, is still alive. "Killed virus" vaccines use a virus that has been killed by heat, chemicals, or other means. Although the virus is dead, it is still able to prime the immune system when it is injected into the body. Among the killed virus vaccines in use today is the Salk vaccine against polio.

Koch hoped to develop a treatment for tuberculosis, and in August 1890, he hinted that he had found a promising substance. This substance, later called tuberculin, was a solution prepared by killing tuberculosis bacteria, then filtering and concentrating the liquid.[14] In November of that year he published a paper in a German medical journal stating that tuberculin might be helpful in diagnosing and curing tuberculosis. In the paper, he said that animals and people with tuberculosis had stronger reactions to this substance than uninfected people, a sign that their immune systems regarded tuberculin and TB bacteria as similar. He also said that tuberculin protected animals from tuberculosis and helped heal tubercles in the lungs. The world beat a path to his door.[15]

The "miracle" substance was headline news in the medical and popular press.[16] Patients besieged Koch's laboratory in Berlin. Other medical centers sent doctors to learn about the treatment. Public demonstrations of the treatment were held. The noted scientist Paul Ehrlich, who had tuberculosis himself, received injections of tuberculin as treatment.[17]

Alas, it soon became clear that this substance, referred to today as "old tuberculin,"[18] did not cure tuberculosis. Within a year, a study showed that only one patient in five was helped by the tuberculin injections, and most of those had a mild form of tuberculosis infecting only the skin.[19]

Even though Koch was deeply embarrassed by the failure of his tuberculin as a cure for TB, the substance did have a useful role to play: It produced a skin reaction in people who had active tuberculosis or who had been infected with tuberculosis in the past (and now had latent tuberculosis infection), so it became useful in diagnosis. Today, we use a very stable derivative of tuberculin called purified protein derivative (PPD) as a diagnostic tool.[20] When PPD is injected just into the skin of someone who has active tuberculosis or latent tuberculosis infection, it produces a round, hard, often red bump within 2 to 3 days. The bump can be measured; it is usually considered positive, meaning that the person is infected, if it is 5 to 10 millimeters or larger (about the size of a dime). This test is called the PPD test or the Mantoux test, for Charles Mantoux, who developed it in 1905, improving on Koch's technique.[21]

Starting around 1900, the quest for a TB vaccine was taken up by two French scientists, Albert Calmette, director of the Pasteur Institute in the city of Lille in northern France, and his research assistant Camille Guérin, a veterinary school graduate. They started with a virulent tuberculosis strain that infected cattle (*Mycobacterium bovis*) and found innovative ways to culture the bacteria. They hoped to weaken the bacteria by "passaging" them from culture to culture, as Pasteur had done with the rabies virus. It was a mammoth task, given TB's sluggish growth rate.

Calmette and Guérin started passaging their cultures in 1906.[22] With astonishing dedication, they transferred the bacteria from one test tube to another every 3 weeks, hoping to weaken the TB bacteria so that they did not cause the disease, but could still evoke a strong enough immune response to protect against it, just as Pasteur's vaccine did against rabies. They worked through World War I, although the city of Lille was mercilessly shelled and fell to the German army in 10 days. By this time, Calmette and Guérin had their vaccine. They then injected it into healthy cows and then injected the cows with virulent bovine tuberculosis bacteria, the original source of the vaccine. Of the nine cows in their experiment, none contracted tuberculosis.

As the war raged on outside the laboratory, Calmette and Guérin continued fighting their own battle, refining the vaccine, transferring ever-weaker strains of bacteria every 3 weeks, for a total of 231 transfers. By 1919 Calmette and Guérin had a weakened form of TB bacteria that had been tested in guinea pigs, rabbits, cattle, and horses.[23] Triumphant, they hoped it would protect people against active TB. The vaccine was called bacille Calmette-Guérin (*bacille* is French for bacillus), soon shortened to BCG.

In 1921, an oral form of the vaccine was given to an infant whose mother had died of TB only hours after giving birth. Because the baby would be cared for by its grandmother, who also had active TB, it was almost certain to become infected and die. The newborn baby received three doses of BCG, and it remained healthy throughout its childhood.[24]

Three years later, Calmette and Guérin gave oral forms of the vaccine to infants and then to adults, with no harm noted. By 1928, well over 100,000 people had received BCG. Despite a disaster in Lubeck, Germany, where children died because they were mistakenly given live tuberculosis bacteria instead of the weakened ones in the vaccine, international organizations and national health services began administering BCG vaccine to young children.[25] Eventually an injectable form was developed, which is still in use today.

In the period of privation after World War II, international agencies began vaccination campaigns using BCG in an attempt to prevent tuberculosis. A few trials of BCG in the 1930s—for example, among nursing students, who were often exposed to patients with active TB—had shown that it reduced TB infections. In the BCG campaign after World War II, nearly 14 million people received the vaccination between 1948 and 1951. Today, BCG is probably the most frequently used vaccine in the world, given as one of the six vaccines in the World Health Organization's expanded program of immunization.

Despite its wide use, it is still not clear how effective BCG is in protecting against TB. A comprehensive review by Dr. George Wills Comstock of Johns Hopkins University, an internationally known TB expert, points out many of the problems:[26]

There are actually many BCG vaccines, not one. Until the mid-1960s, laboratories had to prepare a new culture of BCG every few weeks by taking a sample of the old vaccine and growing it on culture medium to produce more. The method is similar to that used to make sourdough bread, where a piece of the dough is saved and used to raise the next batch of bread. TB bacteria naturally mutate, so the BCG strain may vary from one batch to another and from one laboratory to another. Furthermore, laboratories used different culture media, which might affect the strength of the vaccine. Even when freeze-drying became available in the mid-1960s, laboratories still had to culture some old vaccine in order to make a new lot. The result is that BCG strains around the globe vary in many characteristics.

Furthermore, there was no method for assessing the potency of the vaccine. Many studies did not specify what vaccine was used or what its characteristics were.

Comstock reviewed 19 large clinical trials using BCG to protect against TB. Most of these trials were conducted among people who were thought to be at above-average risk of developing tuberculosis. All the trials had problems. In some trials, people were not given skin tests to diagnose tuberculosis infection before they were vaccinated, so the trials included both people who already had a latent TB infection and so were at high risk for active TB and people who had not been infected. Thus, it was difficult to judge the efficacy of the vaccine in protecting people.

Even when individuals were skin-tested for TB before vaccination, the BCG dose varied from one trial to another. People living in tropical and subtropical regions were more likely to have been infected with other members of the *Mycobacterium* genus, to which TB belongs, because these other mycobacteria were present in their environment. When skin-tested for TB, some of these people had positive skin tests, even though they did not have TB infection. However, everyone with a positive skin test—both those with TB infection and those who had been exposed to other mycobacteria—was excluded from BCG trials, skewing the results.

The BCG vaccine seemed to be more effective in cooler, more temperate regions, where infections with non-TB mycobacteria were uncommon. The closer to the equator the trial was done, apparently the less was the protection provided by BCG.

In several trials there were problems with randomization. For example, the group being vaccinated might have been healthier and more health conscious, because they came to a clinic for vaccination. Other trials never described how people had been allocated to one group or another.

The BCG vaccines used differed from one trial to another. So did the methods of administering them. Some used injection into the skin; others used a multiple-puncture method through the skin. The follow-up methods differed as well. And how long did protection last? That varied, too, in the several different studies, from *no* efficacy after 15 years to about 80 percent after 20 years.

Probably the three best studies of BCG's efficacy were those by the Medical Research Council in Great Britain, by the Public Health Service in the United States, and by Graham Colditz and his colleagues at Harvard.[27] The British study showed a high degree of protection. The U.S. study showed just the opposite: little or no protection. The Colditz study, a meta-analysis that reanalyzed data from many previous studies, suggested that BCG offered about 50 percent protection.

Why are there such discrepancies? One explanation is that the different studies used different strains of BCG, grown in different laboratories, and Peter Small's group at Stanford University has shown that different BCG strains are highly variable genetically, so some strains may have been much more effective than others.

However, the trials usually confirmed that BCG vaccination did protect against miliary and meningeal TB in infants. Miliary TB is disease that spreads like tiny seeds through the body. (The word comes from the Latin *miliaria*, describing the tiny seed of millet, a type of grain.) Meningeal TB (also called tuberculous meningitis) affects the membranes surrounding the spinal cord and the brain and may be deadly in children. Our feeling is that even a very effective strain of BCG does no more than protect infants and very young children against severe forms of TB.

BCG vaccination itself may cause problems. In the past, medical students, nurses, and hospital workers who might have been exposed to TB were sometimes vaccinated with BCG. Usually there was redness and hardening at the site of the injection, which stayed tender for several weeks. In some people—about one-third in a small study—there was ulceration and persistent drainage at the site of the injection.[28] In some patients, usually those with an impaired immune system, a BCG immunization itself might actually disseminate the BCG organisms, with deadly consequences.

Today, "in the United States, the use of BCG vaccination is rarely indicated," says the Centers for Disease Control and Prevention.[29] However, the World Health Organization includes BCG vaccination in its child health immunization program, and many countries eagerly promote BCG vaccination. In Russia, BCG vaccination of all children is vigorously pursued; the vaccine is administered at birth and readministered at age 6 or 7, and then again at age 14 or 15.[30] Yet Russia has a disastrous TB epidemic and has been declared a TB hot spot by the World Health Organization.[31]

Worse than being just ineffective, BCG has a major downside: It makes it difficult for doctors to diagnose active tuberculosis or latent TB infection. At the New Jersey Medical School National Tuberculosis Center, we see many patients from countries where BCG vaccination is common. They may have a cough; they've lost weight; they don't feel well; they come from one of the World Health Organization's TB hot spots. When we do tuberculin skin testing, they have a positive skin reaction. Do they have TB? Or do they just have a positive skin test because they received BCG back home?

There is absolutely no way to tell. Almost all my experience with BCG vaccination, and the experience of many other TB experts, shows that it is worthless in protecting adults. So what do we do? We strongly recommend treating the individual and totally *ignoring* his or her BCG history. If it looks like TB, or latent TB infection, we treat it like TB or latent TB infection. Most authorities support us in this approach. Unfortunately, this approach remains an uphill battle. We are constantly astounded by the blind faith shown in the efficacy of this widely used but poorly effective vaccine by most physicians, who certainly should know better!

BCG has been given to children in most developing countries since the 1920s, including those countries that remain on the World Health Organization's list of hot spots for tuberculosis. Only two countries have never given BCG to their children: the Netherlands and the United States. Today they are among the countries with the very lowest incidence of tuberculosis. So it is fair to say, and most experts agree, that BCG doesn't do much, if anything, to protect adults from TB.

The major advocate for *not* using BCG in the United States is Dr. Comstock, now in his eighties. With carefully conducted studies and projections, and despite great pressure from less informed physicians and from BCG manufacturers, Comstock (who was then with the U.S. Public Health Service) almost single-handedly convinced U.S. health officials not to adopt universal BCG vaccination for children. This was a very prescient move. Although BCG may offer some protection to infants and very young children, the protection clearly does not continue into their adult years, but their positive skin tests usually continue to confuse TB diagnosis.

Because BCG interferes with reading the tuberculin skin test and doesn't protect adults against TB, if it had been widely used in the 1980s and 1990s, it would have masked the resurgence in tuberculosis in the United States that began in 1985 and continued until the early 1990s. We wouldn't have known that we had an epidemic on our hands until much, much later. The national response, which turned the epidemic around, would have been seriously and perhaps fatally delayed.

It is astonishing that scientists have only recently tried to develop new, more effective vaccines for TB. Since 1968, the last BCG trial, vaccines have been developed for measles, mumps, rubella, chicken pox, and many other diseases. Only now, more than 30 years later, are scientists once again taking an interest in developing a vaccine against TB.

Why the lack of interest? No doubt some doctors had a conviction, a gut feeling, that BCG vaccination worked. Many public health organizations and national governments continued to offer BCG vaccination in the belief that they were helping. Since they were convinced that BCG vaccination was a good thing, they thought that it would be sinful to stop using it and stupid to waste money doing yet another huge, expensive 20-year randomized controlled trial. Furthermore, there was an establishment of laboratories manufacturing BCG and health-care workers, doctors, and administrators working in the BCG program, recruiting the patients, giving the vaccine, doing checkups, keeping records. It is very difficult to upset the applecart.

TB rates were declining in industrialized countries, thanks to drugs developed in the 1950s and 1960s. No one saw the need for a better vaccine, which would be most useful in the poorest countries, which could least afford to pay for it, so what was the incentive to develop such a vaccine?

Today, because of heightened ethical concerns, it would probably be impossible to do a study comparing a vaccine to a placebo. A study would have to compare a new vaccine to the best vaccine available. Since such a study would have to be done in Third World countries, where the risk of TB is highest, ethical concerns about informed consent would be complex, as they are with the testing of drugs against AIDS.

Almost a Magic Bullet

In 1910, the world learned that Paul Ehrlich's magic chemical bullet, salvarsan, could cure syphilis. In the 1930s, the search was on to find drugs that would cure other infectious diseases.

When Selman Waksman discovered streptomycin in 1943, it looked like the magic bullet for tuberculosis. Waksman was born into poverty in Ukraine in 1888.[32] His mother nurtured him and encouraged his scholarly interests, but she died soon after he completed his secondary education. Distraught, Waksman emigrated to America and went to live with a cousin who owned a farm in New Jersey. Looking for a university where he could continue his education—one that he could afford—he approached another Russian immigrant, Professor Jacob Lipman at nearby Rutgers College.

Waksman worked on the farm and at odd jobs around the college to earn his keep while he studied under Lipman. His particular interest was a group of soil microbes called actinomycetes. After getting his advanced degrees, he moved to California. During World War II he was called upon to aid the war effort. His expertise in soil microbes was needed to prevent the bottoms of ships from being fouled by marine organisms and to protect American soldiers and their equipment from the fungi in the jungles of the South Pacific.

His war work protecting ships, soldiers, and equipment from environmental microorganisms led Waksman to become interested in antibiotics, microorganisms like penicillin that kill other microorganisms. In fact, he coined the word *antibiotic*,[33] now one of the most important words in the medical lexicon. After the war he moved back to his laboratory in the New Jersey Agricultural Experiment Station at Rutgers University and had funding from major drug companies that wanted to find new antibiotics. His son, a medical student, suggested that he look for an antibiotic that would work against tuberculosis.

As chance would have it, an actinomycete had recently been isolated from the throat of a sick chicken by a scientist at a New Jersey agricultural station.[34] The chicken had probably picked up the microbe from pecking about in the soil looking for food, as chickens do. (The microbe was not a cause of the chicken's sickness; it was an accidental but fortuitous finding.) Two graduate students, Albert Schatz and Elizabeth Bugie, worked hard to identify the organism: *Streptomyces griseus*. From it they then isolated a substance with new antibiotic properties. In only a few months they learned that this substance, which they called streptomycin, killed organisms like tuberculosis bacteria that were not affected by other new antibiotics. In 1952, Waksman received the Nobel Prize for the discovery of streptomycin. Schatz and Bugie, who had done all the work, were not acknowledged, and to this day Schatz has remained, rightfully, exceptionally bitter, even though his name was on the patent. Bugie, according to her daughter Patricia, was told "some day you'll get married and have a family and it's not important that your name be on the patent." Bugie said, "If women's lib had been around, my name would have been on the patent." Schatz recalled that 80 percent of the royalties from streptomycin went to a foundation at Rutgers, 10 percent to Waksman, 2 percent to Schatz, and 0.22 percent to Bugie. Bugie died in 2001. In 1943, TB experts at the Mayo Clinic in Minnesota heard about Waksman's work and began to collaborate with him on animal experiments, with much success. Then a woman known to this day only as Patricia—Patricia T in some accounts, Patricia S in others—came to their attention. Just 21, she was dying of tuberculosis at a Minnesota sanatorium. She weighed 75 pounds. She had had surgery on one lung, but her tuberculosis had spread to the other lung, usually a lethal consequence. As she had no other chance, her doctors suggested that she be the first person to get experimental treatment with streptomycin. Between November 1944 and early 1945 she received many painful injections of streptomycin, with the later injections containing higher concentrations of the drug. Patricia returned from the brink of death, left the hospital, got married, and had three children. She may still be alive today.

Imagine the headlines that this miraculous cure prompted. It would be like waking up today and reading "Cancer Cure Discovered," "Heart Disease Conquered," or "Drug Cures AIDS!" It was delirious, wonderful news.

More Miracles Needed

Streptomycin was indeed a miracle drug, but it wasn't enough, as doctors, researchers, and patients discovered all too soon. Patients got better, but then many of them relapsed. The tuberculosis bacteria were fighting back.

Tuberculosis bacteria are notoriously difficult to kill. They stick together in their hard-coated clumps like the shield wall of Roman soldiers. The coating is nearly impenetrable to antibiotics, so it is very difficult for them to reach the bacteria in the core. Even when a drug like streptomycin manages to break through, some bacteria are innately resistant. When an antibiotic kills off the vulnerable bacteria, the resistant ones survive and multiply. Within a single tuberculosis cavity in the lung, there are hundreds of millions of TB bacteria. As they multiply, some mutate and become resistant to the antibiotic.

It soon became clear that instead of just one drug, a multipronged approach was needed: an antibiotic that would kill off the vulnerable bacteria, and another one—or two or three—that could kill off the bacteria that had mutated and so had survived the first drug. Doctors needed something analogous to the multibladed razors advertised on TV, where the first blade cuts off most of the hairs, then a second and a third blade cut off the hairs that were missed by the first.

Many things can go wrong with antibiotic treatment if it is not done carefully and correctly. The doctor may prescribe only one or two drugs when four or five are needed. The antibiotics may be given at too low a dose. The patient may not take the full dose or may skip doses. The medication may be poorly manufactured so that it is not absorbed or does not contain enough of the active ingredient.

The most important principle of drug treatment is that TB bacteria are most vulnerable at the outset. At that point, they can be killed off relatively easily by simple, cheap, effective antibiotics. Once these antibiotics have been misused, however, whether by the doctor or by the patient, the bacteria become resistant and much more difficult to combat. This is how the current worldwide epidemic of multi-drug-resistant tuberculosis was created. Surprisingly, most often it is the doctor, not the patient, who is at fault.

Once created, multi-drug-resistant strains spread just the same way as ordinary TB—through the air—resulting in a human-made disease that, ultimately, few if any antibiotics can cure.

Drug Miracles, for Now

Soon after streptomycin was introduced, scientists found other new drugs that would kill the TB bacteria. After streptomycin, introduced for clinical use in 1946, came *para*-aminosalicylic acid (PAS) in 1946, isoniazid in 1952, pyrazinamide in 1952, ethambutol in 1963, and rifampin in 1966. To this day, isoniazid and rifampin remain our most powerful drugs against TB, even though they were discovered 35 and 50 years ago. Drug companies have come up with new combinations and variations, but there has been no new class of drugs against TB since 1966.

When these drugs were first introduced, patients had to take three of them every day for 18 to 24 months. Then, when the powerful oral drug rifampin was introduced, the length of treatment could be shortened to 9 months, although patients still had to take 5 pills every day. For the patient, of course, even nine months of daily pill taking seemed like a very long time, particularly since he or she usually began to feel better after a few weeks. Then scientists at the British Medical Research Council came up with a brilliant idea: they showed that if the patient was given one of the earliest TB drugs, pyrazinamide, along with isoniazid and rifampin for the first 2 months, treatment could be shortened to a mere 6 months. Doctors called the 6-month or 9-month treatment "short course," but it seemed shorter for the doctors than for the patients.

Even so, for patients who just a few years previously had had only a 50–50 chance of surviving tuberculosis, short-course treatment was miraculous. If they took their medications, they would feel better within a few weeks. They would no longer be infectious. Their families, friends, and colleagues would be safe. They could continue to work and follow their daily routines. However, they had to keep taking the drugs faithfully, even though they felt well, in order to kill any lingering bacteria, which, if not entirely eliminated, could cause relapse and often did.

With powerful, effective new drug regimens to treat TB, a new era in TB treatment began. It was time to reevaluate some deeply entrenched strategies—the sanatoriums, the enforced bed rest, treatment in the open air, and devastating surgery. Long-term hospitalization became a thing of the past. There wasn't any reason to keep sanatoriums open, and the sanatorium industry began to shut down.

Closing the Sans

In 1974 I became director of the Pulmonary Division of what is now the University of Medicine and Dentistry of New Jersey, New Jersey Medical School. I was the new guy in town. Although I was a relatively experienced pulmonologist and TB physician and the former director of the Bureau of Tuberculosis for the New York City Department of Health, I was thought to have little political baggage in my new job. So I was asked to chair a task force considering the fate of the New Jersey State Hospital for Chest Diseases at Glen Gardner, the State TB Sanitorium. I had already survived a media blitz as head of TB in New York when I closed the TB unit at Sea View Hospital on Staten Island, which was established in 1829 as a poor farm and hospital, became New York City's TB hospital, and was the place where isoniazid was first shown to provide rapid cures for desperately ill patients.

When word got out that we were considering closing the Glen Gardner sanatorium in New Jersey, there were protests and headlines. We met stiff resistance. Huge TB sanatoriums were major local employers, often providing many patronage jobs. Some even had taxing power in their local towns. To be as objective as possible, my task force visited every one of the 173 patients who were then hospitalized at Glen Gardner. We found that more than three-quarters—133 individuals—needed only careful outpatient care. Of the other 40, there were 2 who needed short-term hospital care, 2 who needed long-term hospital care, 28 who needed nursing home care, and 8 who needed care in a psychiatric hospital. Our task force unanimously recommended closing the sanatorium and transferring the patients to more appropriate care. For most of them, outpatient treatment was more humane and would allow them to lead more normal lives with their families.

There was a huge uproar. One newspaper headline boldly stated, "Some Will Die."

But we were able to justify our recommendation that the hospital be closed, an action that would not only give more humane and appropriate care but save New Jersey $3 million annually. In what was an unprecedented move at the time, we recommended that one-third of the money saved be transferred to a different state agency to fund an improved outpatient system to handle the patients who previously would have been hospitalized in the sanatorium.

TB—Almost Gone

In the 1970s and early 1980s, tuberculosis rates were going down all over the United States. Eliminating tuberculosis domestically was within the nation's grasp. Since nobody was concerned about international TB, everyone was confident that with another few dollars and another few years of effort, the job would be done. But that last, crucial step was never taken. Things went wrong.

During the Nixon administration, members of Congress were given the idea that declining tuberculosis rates meant that tuberculosis was a disease of the past. They were tragically wrong. In 1971, when I was still director of the Bureau of Tuberculosis of the New York City Health Department, I went to Washington and testified before the House Subcommittee on Public Health and Environment along with a number of other experts. Congress was considering a bill that would end earmarked funding for tuberculosis and convert the money into "block grants" that states could use for whatever purposes they wished.

I pointed out that tuberculosis was a well-understood disease and the only one of the then top 20 causes of death in the United States that was totally curable. I said that essentially the treatments were known and effective. We could eliminate TB with just a little more effort. "But," I said, "the delivery of the fruits of such research to those citizens, usually the poor and the disadvantaged most in need of it, is clearly deficient." I pointed out that even then the number of cases of TB had increased in Brooklyn and that the rate in Harlem was more than five times higher than the rate in the city as a whole. I argued that the federal administration was wrong in arguing that state funds could fill the gap, with help from the vague federal block grants. My argument was that the states, with their new-found freedom, would spend the money for their own political priorities, not to eliminate TB.

Finally, I told the congressional committee, "Unless other funding is found, New York City faces an unparalleled health crisis resulting in the closing of our eight combined chest clinics which give comprehensive care to 6500 complicated tuberculosis patients. The result clearly will be a decrease in tuberculosis surveillance, requirement for longer hospital stays, and ultimately a reversal in the downward trends in this disease that we have all been so proud of."

I was a voice in the wilderness. Block grants came in. Funding for TB was drastically cut or eliminated. Across the country, TB rates began to climb. And an unprecedented epidemic broke out in New York City.

4

TB in the Time of AIDS

When Dr. Reynard McDonald says, "I've never seen it before," I listen. Like me, McDonald trained under the legendary Dr. Julia Jones, a passionate and powerful TB mentor, at Harlem Hospital, ground zero for tuberculosis back when we were residents in the late 1960s. He had seen a lot of things since then.

McDonald and I had just examined a desperately ill patient in the pulmonary disease unit, which I headed, at the New Jersey Medical School University Hospital in Newark. It was sometime in 1981. The patient had several abscesses in his brain caused by tuberculosis. McDonald said, "This is extremely rare. We're seeing all these people with weird forms of tuberculosis that I have never seen before."

Tuberculosis usually attacks the upper part of the lung. In industrialized countries, only about 15 percent of TB is extrapulmonary, or outside the lungs. (Extrapulmonary TB was much more common in the past, and it still is in the Third World; no one knows why.) When TB attacks the brain and the central nervous system, it usually causes meningitis, an inflammation of the membranes around the brain and spinal cord. But our patient had multiple large abscesses in his brain that clearly were not meningitis. They looked almost like tumors.

McDonald's comments were eye-opening. As we stopped to talk in the hallway, he told me that he had recently begun to see a huge increase in extrapulmonary TB—tuberculosis of the wrist, of the spine, of the lymph nodes, of the intestine, of the rectum, of the sack of membranes around the heart, even of the testicles. And now, of course, there was our patient with tuberculosis of the brain. He had noticed that this "weird TB," as he called it, was appearing in gay men and in injecting drug users. It looked to him as if these patients all had the new syndrome that people were then calling gay-related immunodeficiency (GRID). Soon, the problem got a more accurate name. Instead of GRID, which incorrectly and insensitively focused on only one risk group or transmission category, the disorder came to be called acquired immunodeficiency syndrome (AIDS), and it soon was clear that its cause was human immunodeficiency virus (HIV). Because HIV destroys the immune system, people infected with HIV are vulnerable to diseases like TB, which occur more often in them than in people with healthy immune systems.

But we didn't know all this back then. Nor did we know whom HIV infected or how to diagnose it. Doctors had known for a long time that TB was more common in people with suppressed immune systems, such as those who received immunosuppressive drugs in cancer chemotherapy or those who received steroids to control asthma, arthritis, and other kinds of inflammation. What McDonald was seeing seemed to make sense in that context, but it was still very strange. No one knew why so many people suddenly seemed to have weakened immune systems, especially because so many of them were young. The normal immune system gets weaker with age, but these patients were in their twenties and thirties.

I said, "Well, if these strange cases of TB are now occurring in these newly described immunodeficient patients, you've got a new syndrome. You'd better start collecting the cases, and we'll see how the pieces fit together." With the help of one of our pulmonary fellows, Dr. Gnana Sunderam, we made a presentation at the annual joint meeting of the American Thoracic Society and the American Lung Association in Miami in May 1984. An abstract of our presentation was published in a medical journal, then called the *American Review of Respiratory Diseases*, in April 1984.[1]

Our study was the first to report that this new disease, which by this time was being called AIDS, was fueling the latent fire of a familiar old infection, with strange presentations of tuberculosis. The first American cases of AIDS had been reported in 1981 in *Morbidity and Mortality Weekly Report*, the ominously named publication of the U.S. Centers for Disease Control (CDC). We had no idea then how serious this dreadful synergy between AIDS and TB would become.

Our presentation, with its unexpected results and conclusions about this weird form of TB, was greeted with skepticism. Doctors at the Miami meeting asked if these uncommon presentations of TB might be caused by other mycobacteria that were known to infect people with weakened immune systems, such as *Mycobacterium avium-intracellulare*, or even by a different bug, *Pneumocystis carinii*. The questioners were on the right track. People with normal immune systems usually have ordinary TB. But we reasoned that in a patient with a weakened immune system, TB might take on unfamiliar forms. Essentially, without a strong army of macrophages to contain the TB bacteria in the lungs, the infection is free to roam throughout the body. We just hadn't seen this happen much until AIDS came on the scene. Besides, the other bugs the questioners mentioned, though they do cause opportunistic infections in AIDS patients, are mild compared to TB. Opportunistic infections, by definition, become dangerous only in people with severely weakened immune systems (hence the name opportunistic—they take advantage of this opportunity). TB, however, isn't an opportunistic infection. It is always strong enough to cause disease, whether one's immune system is weak or strong. A strong bug like TB is called a pathogen.

Sunderam, McDonald, and I went on collecting cases of these strange forms of TB, and a year later we wrote up our first 29 cases for publication and submitted the article to the *Journal of the American Medical Association* (*JAMA*). Like all other respected medical journals, *JAMA* sends articles out for "peer review" before it accepts them for publication. We said in our paper that we had no idea why we were seeing so much tuberculosis in injecting drug users. I was quite surprised and even embarrassed when one of the anonymous reviewers wrote, "That's in the literature," and referred to a paper I myself had written with Dr. Charles Felton (of Harlem Hospital) and Dr. John Edsall (now of Columbia-Presbyterian) in 1979.[2]

I had clean forgotten about our old paper, which described an extremely high rate of tuberculosis in injecting drug users. In fact, we had found that injecting drug users were more than six times as likely to have active tuberculosis as patients in Harlem Hospital who were not drug users. The tuberculosis rate in central Harlem was high, as might be expected in a very poor neighborhood, but it was nothing like the rate we had found in the injecting drug users. We had concluded that drug dependence itself was a risk factor for tuberculosis, although we did not have any idea how drug dependence impaired the immune system. Possibly some of these drug users had unrecognized HIV infection; our study was done before HIV/AIDS had been identified and years before there was an AIDS test. Or perhaps some contaminant of the drugs they injected, such as talc, made their lungs susceptible to TB. We will never know, but in any case, we recommended that patients in methadone treatment programs who had positive skin tests for tuberculosis be given the TB preventive drug isoniazid when they came to receive their daily methadone. In a methadone clinic, a clinic worker watches while each addict takes his or her methadone, usually swallowing it dissolved in an orange drink. We didn't realize it back in 1979, but we were suggesting a precursor for directly observed therapy (DOT), now a powerful tool in the treatment of TB. As is usual when someone suggests an unconventional idea, this too was ignored. Maybe that's why I had forgotten the paper.

JAMA published our paper on unusual forms of TB in injecting drug users with AIDS in 1986.[3] As an extension of our earlier abstract, it was the first study linking HIV/AIDS to tuberculosis. We had studied 136 adults with AIDS over a period of $3^{1}/_{2}$ years, and 29 of them (21 percent) had severe and unusual forms of tuberculosis.

Soon we had an additional group of nine more cases, each weirder than the last. All of these patients had HIV infection or AIDS, and their TB affected the central nervous system, which was most unusual.[4] The trend continued. Of the 420 patients with AIDS whom we had seen by late 1986, 52 (or 12 percent) had tuberculosis, and in 10 of those 52 (or 19 percent), tuberculosis affected the brain or spinal cord.

We were learning to be suspicious in diagnosing these patients. In ordinary circumstances, a positive tuberculin skin test indicates past or present latent tuberculosis infection, so most patients with active TB are assumed to have a positive skin test. But 27 of the 29 TB patients in our first report had negative skin tests. The tuberculin skin test measures a reaction to tuberculin by the patient's immune system, but these patients' immune systems were obviously so depleted by HIV that they couldn't muster a response to the tuberculin test.[5] We had to order more aggressive tests, such as biopsies and blood cultures, to confirm the diagnosis of any TB that we suspected.

As we saw case after case, we realized that something exceedingly unusual was going on and that we were part of a larger search for answers. Before and during the time we were collecting our strange cases of TB, other physicians were reporting cases of the new disease AIDS from Miami and Haiti and New York and San Francisco. Doctors were learning about AIDS as they went along. It became clear that the first groups it devastated were gay men and injecting drug users, and then their sex partners and their children.

The AIDS epidemic didn't hit the headlines and get attention in the centers of power until the actor Rock Hudson died and Randy Shilts wrote his highly acclaimed book *And the Band Played On*. Shilts described "Patient Zero," a promiscuous male flight attendant who infected many others during the "Operation Sail" celebration of the two hundredth birthday of the United States in 1976. I don't like to think of using someone who is ill with a deadly disease as a "Patient Zero" or as a "poster child" in appealing for help or attention. But the fact was that TB needed somebody like that. This disease, which had always been a serious global problem, had been preventable and curable for three decades, but nonetheless was spreading throughout the world, fueled by the frightening companion epidemic called AIDS.

Soon we had our poster child, a middle-class man from a small city in upstate New York.

Storm Rising

In late summer and early fall, people who live on the East Coast of the United States or along the Gulf of Mexico watch their television sets very carefully and listen to their news radio stations for distant early warnings of hurricanes that may destroy their homes and their cities and threaten their lives. In 1991, we were in the midst of our own hurricane season, but we were watching for a different sort of storm, one that would prove far more devastating than any wind off the sea. We didn't have long to wait.

For me, Saturday mornings are usually quiet. I spend them doing ordinary chores: taking the car to the gas station, going to the supermarket and the dry cleaner, tackling all the mail that's piled up on the coffee table. On this Saturday morning, November 16, 1991, right there on the front page of the *New York Times* (just below the fold) was a story by Robert McFadden: "A Drug-Resistant TB Results in 13 Deaths in New York Prisons."[6]

To my mind this single newspaper article proved to be as notable in its own way as Koch's discovery of the tubercle bacillus in 1882 or the first use of antibiotics in the fight against TB in the middle of the twentieth century. For the first time ever, pundits, policy makers, politicians, as well as ordinary people were forced to take notice of something that previously had concerned only a minuscule cadre of TB doctors and a few public health officials.

Most people remember that story as the one about "the Syracuse prison guard who died," although it actually reported that 12 inmates and a guard had died from multi-drug-resistant strains of tuberculosis. One of the reasons TB gets no respect as a major killer is that it is invisible to the mainstream. It seems to most often strike people who are homeless or who live in poverty. Even though they live in the same society as the prosperous, sharing the air with everyone around them—doctors, bankers, lawyers, teachers, workers on the assembly line, people at the coffee machine, people on the bus or subway or airplane—nobody notices the homeless or the desperately poor.

People noticed the guard. Who cared about prisoners? They had committed crimes; that's why they were in prison. But the guard—he was one of us: a white, middle-class, middle-aged man working in the civil service.

He was dedicated; he even continued to come to work while he was under-going treatment for cancer. In fact, he was guarding inmates who were being treated for multi-drug-resistant tuberculosis in a hospital in Syracuse. The guard's immune system was weakened because of his cancer treatment. The inmates, from one of whom he caught multi-drug-resistant tuberculosis, all had weakened immune systems because they were infected with HIV.

The 12 inmates in McFadden's article came from two separate prisons, and no one from either group had ever been within miles of anyone from the other group. Eight had been at a correctional facility in New York City that had about 1000 inmates and 250 employees; they died at St. Clare's Hospital in New York City. The other four were from the Auburn Correctional Facility in upstate New York, a maximum-security prison with 1700 inmates and a staff of over 700; they died at the nearby University Hospital of the State University of New York in Syracuse, where the prison guard had been watching them.

There was more bad news: Although the prison outbreaks in New York City and in Syracuse were separated by hundreds of miles, they were caused by the same strain of multi-drug-resistant TB. Strains of TB, like those of other organisms, have distinctive DNA fingerprints. (This is discussed fur-ther in Chapter 8, "Fingerprinting the Bacteria.") A molecular biologist can distinguish the strain that causes the disease in Joe Smith from the strain that causes the disease in Bill Jones—or discover that Smith and Jones have the same strain. Or even find that Smith has the strain common in San Francisco, and Jones has the strain common in Siberia.

But the four inmates in Syracuse and the eight in New York City had never been in contact. So how could they all have had the same deadly strain of multi-drug-resistant tuberculosis? Since prison inmates are often moved around from prison to prison (sometimes to thwart the formation of gangs) an unidentified inmate or inmates probably had spread the multi-drug-resistant strain through the system as they were transferred. Those uniden-tified inmates were probably still somewhere in the system, continuing to spread the disease to other prisoners. Or they might have been released and be at home with family and friends, spreading the disease in the community.

The New York State commissioner of corrections, Thomas A. Coughlin, III, told the New York Times that 84 cases of tuberculosis had been identi-fied among the state's 60,000 prisoners. He said that it wasn't clear how many of the TB cases were drug resistant, but that the multi-drug-resistant strain was a "deadly threat" to the other 60,000 prisoners in the state's 68 prisons and to the 28,000 people who were employed in the prison system, and by extension to their families and communities.[7]

The New York State Health Department decided that all current prison inmates, all new inmates, and all prison employees were to undergo mandatory testing for TB every year. The same *New York Times* story quoted Dr. George DiFerdinando, Jr., then director of the New York State Health Department's TB control program, as saying, "We're going to control it in the prisons, where it's easiest to control. But the real question is how are you going to control it now that it is established in the community?" The Syracuse prison guard, infected with the multi-drug-resistant TB that ultimately killed him, continued to go home to his family every night, as did the nurses, secretaries, cooks, guards, clerks, and other prison employees.

The *Times* story was just the beginning. The next day, McFadden reported that another prison inmate had died from TB in the Syracuse hospital and that the same multi-drug-resistant TB strain had been identified a few months before in outbreaks in hospitals in New York and Miami, where HIV and AIDS were flourishing.[8] A five-part *New York Times* series about tuberculosis followed, with the first three parts appearing above the fold. There were front-page stories in New York's tabloid newspapers as well, and a *Newsweek* cover story. The network morning talk shows gave the story extensive coverage, as did the *McNeil-Lehrer News Hour.* (Ted Koppel's *Nightline* had already run a program on the connection between multi-drug-resistant TB and HIV several months earlier, in June 1991.) Because of the tragic death of one white middle-aged man, the Syracuse prison guard, more attention was paid to TB in just a few months than any of us had seen in our entire careers battling this disease

A Double-Edged Sword

We knew that HIV infection or AIDS weakens the immune system and makes people at least 800 times more likely to have their latent TB infection activated. It wasn't realized until later that the reverse is also true: Active tuberculosis further suppresses the immune system of AIDS patients; curing tuberculosis actually improves the immune system.

The lethal combination of AIDS and TB is a worldwide problem. According to the Joint *United Nations Program on HIV/AIDS* (UNAIDS), at the beginning of 2000 there were 34.6 million people in the world who were infected with HIV.[9] In the countries where most AIDS patients live, TB is the most prevalent serious infection. One-third of the people who are reported as dying of AIDS actually die of TB. Worldwide, TB is the *leading* killer of people with HIV/AIDS. We who take care of AIDS patients know that essentially nobody actually dies of AIDS. AIDS weakens the immune system; people with AIDS die of diseases that are shrugged off by people with healthy immune systems.

In the early 1990s, in sub-Saharan Africa, Haiti, and Asia, the majority of adults already had latent tuberculosis infections. The TB bacteria were in their bodies, but their immune systems were keeping the bacteria in check. When AIDS came on the scene and destroyed these people's immune systems, a waiting TB epidemic exploded. In several African countries, from 20 to 67 percent of patients with tuberculosis were also infected with AIDS. Autopsy studies in some west African countries showed that tuberculosis was the most frequent concurrent infection in patients who died of AIDS.[10] They had AIDS, but they died of tuberculosis.

The situation is no better today. In some countries in Africa, 20 to 30 percent of pregnant women are infected with HIV, a sign of what HIV/AIDS is doing to the young, productive, economically active population. In South Africa, the most economically developed and sophisticated country south of the Sahara, 20 percent of the population is infected with HIV. Probably one-third to one-half of the people in these countries also have latent TB infection. In the countries with the largest number of people with HIV/AIDS, TB is still the most common cause of death in AIDS patients. This is particularly tragic because even in patients with AIDS, TB remains preventable and curable.

The co-existence and dreadful synergy between TB and HIV/AIDS is well known to international health-care experts and to nurses and doctors working in affected communities. They see daily the tragic burden these dual epidemics place on young families, especially in Africa and Asia.

Therefore, I am constantly amazed that there is not more collegiality and cooperation among the legions of professionals involved with each disease, from social workers to doctors and nurses to researchers, donors, and government officials. For some reason, over the years, major AIDS meetings, such as the International Conference on AIDS, have only rarely included high-profile plenary sessions on TB. This may be a symptom, reflecting perhaps, an arrogant mind-set among some AIDS professionals. These professionals seem to prefer to deal with AIDS while ignoring the companion epidemic of TB.

It isn't entirely clear why this is so. At the beginning of the HIV/AIDS epidemic in industrialized nations, the first patients—young, gay men—were unlikely to have latent TB infection and thus usually became sick with other organisms. Furthermore, they were often considered (without any scientific basis) to be more likely to adhere to their treatment regimens. This group was considered very different from the other major transmission category, injecting drug users, who usually had very high latent TB infection rates and, therefore, more active TB. Injecting drug users were often considered far less adherent and more difficult to deal with (again, without any scientific basis).

Perhaps the lack of cooperation and communication among these health professionals may have occurred because, historically, at least in industrialized nations, TB patients were usually cared for by pulmonary physicians or public health clinics, and AIDS patients were usually cared for by infectious disease physicians.

One seasoned observer, Nance Monot-Upham, is an economist, journalist, activist, and consultant to the International Union Against Tuberculosis and Lung Disease. For more than a decade she has been promoting the wisdom of controlling TB and HIV/AIDS in context with each other through a nongovernmental organization, SIDALERT (SIDA = AIDS in French), which had 450 volunteers and 14 paid staff. With funds largely from the European Union she published a widely circulated newsletter addressing the TB-HIV synergy and interaction in Africa. Monot-Upham feels that AIDS patients, and thus their governments or NGOs, feared being stigmatized with the more easily transmissible TB. She thinks that the resulting pressure to separate AIDS and TB caused many tensions and gradually led donors to pull out of funding for her NGO.

Because tuberculosis is spread through the air by breathing, rather than specific risk behavior, obviously it represents a much greater health threat to the world's population (more in developing countries than in industrialized ones) than HIV/AIDS. Yet, paradoxically tuberculosis still receives relatively little attention from U.N. agencies (aside from WHO) and advocacy groups, compared to HIV/AIDS.

However, it is clear to me that health experts increasingly recognize the interaction between TB and HIV/AIDS. They see that curing or preventing TB increases or preserves immune function and that TB treatments such as directly observed therapy are now frequently being studied for complex AIDS treatment regimens. Ultimately the groups fighting each disease must cooperate more closely to prevent further loss of life. The recent global effort to consider a "Massive Effort to Fight Diseases of Poverty" (TB, HIV/AIDS, and malaria), now called the Global Health Fund and endorsed by the WHO and some (but certainly not all) nongovernmental agencies (with varying degrees of enthusiasm), is encouraging, suggesting that cooperation might come sooner rather than later. Monot-Upham quotes a high South African official: "Let's control TB which is preventable and curable, so we can address ourselves to HIV/AIDS in the manner it deserves." May this occur, and soon!

End of the Evil Empire

At about the same time the Syracuse prison guard died of TB, an event that seemed to be totally unrelated occurred: The Soviet Union fell apart. By the end of 1991, the USSR no longer existed. The former Soviet states had declared their freedom and become independent countries, of which Russia was the largest. It was as if the Confederates had won the Civil War in the United States and the nation had split.

The sudden disintegration of the Soviet Union put the Russian economy (and those of the countries that had formerly been part of the Soviet Union) through what the Russians called "shock therapy" and international economists called a "meltdown." People didn't get paid; supplies didn't get through; the system stopped working. Unemployment, social disruption, and alcoholism led to disarray in the health-care system. Age-adjusted mortality rose by almost 33 percent between 1990 and 1994; that meant that the average citizen had a one-third greater chance of dying. Life expectancy declined for the first time ever recorded in an industrialized country in peacetime. Russian men could expect to live only to 58, whereas they had previously lived to almost 64. Russian women could expect to live to 71 instead of 74. At the same time, life expectancy in the United States was increasing.[11]

Why were Russians dying so much earlier? The main reasons for the increased mortality were cardiovascular diseases, injuries, infectious diseases such as pneumonia and influenza, chronic liver disease and other problems related to alcoholism, and cancer. Malnutrition was common and still is. "Kids in the military are dying of hunger and malnutrition. Basic supplies are lacking," said Russian-American journalist Masha Gessen in February 2000.[12] In such an unhealthy population, it was no surprise that AIDS, syphilis, drug addiction, alcoholism, and TB increased. TB incidence increased by 28 percent, reaching 85 cases per 100,000 in 1999.[13]

American demographer Murray Feshbach of Georgetown University in Washington, D.C., has predicted that the Russian population will decline from 148 million in 1990 to 138 million or lower in 2015, "given anticipated higher mortality rates as losses from the epidemics of tuberculosis and AIDS manifest themselves after 2005."[14] He believes that the population might fall to 80 million—scarcely more than half its current number—by 2050.

Tuberculosis began its astonishing upward surge in Russia in 1991, just as the Soviet Union fell apart. From the lowest point it had ever reached in

Russia, 34 cases per 100,000 in the civilian population in 1991 (compared to 10.1 per 100,000 in the United States), the TB rate shot upward to 82 cases per 100,000 in 1997,[15] 85 cases per 100,000 in 1999 (compared to 6.4 per 100,000 in the United States), and today it is even higher. Several regions reported a doubling of TB death rates. By 1994, Russia had the highest TB death rate in Europe, and 40 percent of the victims were people younger than 39, who should have been in their most productive years.[16]

At the same time, petty crime was increasing, and the Russians were jailing more people than ever. The United States once led the world in the number of its citizens imprisoned, but by 1998 Russia had taken over the lead, imprisoning about 700 people per 100,000.[17] In some regions today, 1000 of every 100,000 people are imprisoned—in other words, one person in every hundred is a prisoner. The State Administration for the Carrying Out of Punishment (called GUIN, from its initials in Russian), a division of the Russian Ministry of Justice, is in charge of the prison system, which now holds more than 1 million inmates. Most are men, and many are young: 29 percent are under age 25.[18]

Conditions in Russian prisons are far worse than those in the deteriorating civilian economy outside the prison walls. The prisons are vastly overcrowded, crammed with two or three times as many prisoners as they were designed for. About 1 prisoner in 10 has active, infectious TB, which spreads easily to other prisoners in the crowded quarters. TB rates in Russian prisons are 40 to 50 times higher than those in the civilian population.[19] Visitors and prison staff are also exposed and carry the risk home at night to their families.

About 300,000 prisoners are released from Russian prisons every year, either after having served their sentences or through amnesties, which are sometimes proclaimed to relieve overcrowding or to release prisoners who are ill. In addition to the 10 percent who have active tuberculosis,[20] more than 80 percent of the released prisoners have been infected with latent TB. Each of these has a 1 in 10 chance of developing active, infectious TB sometime in his lifetime. Many of these released prisoners have been infected with multi-drug-resistant TB.

Every year, the released prisoners are replaced by another 300,000 people entering the Russian prison system. They may be healthy when they enter, but when they spin out the revolving door, almost all of them will carry tuberculosis with them since active, transmissible TB is so prevalent. Because of the high prevalence of multi-drug-resistance, many of those newly infected will carry multi-drug-resistant organisms.

The Missing Ingredient: HIV

The growing tuberculosis epidemic in Russian prisons was a timebomb wait-ing to explode. It would become something far, far worse than anyone in that fairly well run prison in Syracuse could have imagined. The untold part of this story, which makes it a harbinger of disaster for Russia and possibly for the rest of the world, is that these sky-high rates of tuberculosis in Russia and Russian prisons were occurring *in the almost total absence of HIV/AIDS infection.* When Russia entered the 1990s, it did not have many cases of HIV and AIDS, compared with much of the rest of the world. But it was just a matter of time before it did.

When Communism fell, rates of sexually transmitted diseases rocketed upward. Poor and hungry women turned to prostitution. New cases of syphilis increased by 77 times between 1990 and 1999. For young girls aged only 10 to 14, rates of syphilis increased by 50 times. About 40 percent of Russian prostitutes, who often use intravenous drugs, are now infected with HIV.[21] An alarming number of young men being drafted into the army are rejected because of syphilis.[22]

At the same time, intravenous drug use also rocketed upward. Cheap heroin from Afghanistan and Tajikistan flooded into Russia in the late 1990s. Drug use, like alcoholism, became a way to deal with unemployment and everyday despair. In Russia, intravenous drug use is probably the major route for HIV infection. For example, there was an outbreak of HIV among intravenous drug users in the Siberian city of Irkutsk, where, according to the *New York Times,* AIDS cases and drug addiction went from almost zero to an official count of 5000 new cases of AIDS and 8500 drug addicts in 1 year. Experts thought the actual numbers could be ten times higher.[23] In Russia as a whole, there are about 2 million intravenous drug users, accord-ing to an expert quoted by the *New York Times* in April 2000. The HIV/AIDS virus spreads among them through shared needles and methods used to prepare drug solutions.[24]

In just the first 9 months of 1999, 12,000 new cases of HIV were reported, and 90 percent of them were in intravenous drug users, said Deputy Health Minister Gennady Onishchenko, as reported by the *Moscow Times.* The Ministry of Health reported that Russia had 23,502 people with HIV infection by November 1999, but an AIDS expert, Vadim Pokrovsy, told the *Moscow Times* that the real number was at least 100,000 and per-haps 200,000.[25]

The most recent World Health Organization report on AIDS noted that injecting drug use in Russia was fueling the world's steepest increase in

AIDS.[26] The number of people with HIV infection in the states of the former Soviet Union doubled between 1997 and 1999. In these states and the other countries of central and eastern Europe, HIV infections rose by more than a third in one year, 1999. The World Health Organization's report went on to give some appalling details. In Moscow and surrounding towns, three to five times as many HIV infections were recorded in the first 9 months of 1999 as in all previous years combined. Injecting drug use was becoming common, not just in Moscow, but in many cities in Russia and Ukraine. And injecting drug use was occurring not just among unemployed young adults, but even among children under the age of 14.

Projections suggest that Russia will have 1 million HIV-infected people by 2003, and that 12 percent of the population—more than 17 million people—will be infected by 2015. Until now, HIV was the missing ingredient in the Russian tuberculosis epidemic. Now it's here, an appalling, rapidly growing monster that is inevitably adding powerful fuel to the Russian tuberculosis disaster.

No Man Is an Island

Americans were not concerned about tuberculosis in prisoners in Syracuse until they spread it to one of "us," a member of the middle class, the prison guard. Why, then, should they be concerned about tuberculosis in Russia?

People travel. There are 7 million airplane flights a year, carrying about 500 million passengers. Some 50 million people visit the United States each year. Nearly 700,000 legal immigrants come to live in the United States every year, and the nation harbors an estimated 7.1 to 9 million illegal immigrants. The vast majority of immigrants, both legal and illegal, come from countries where TB is common. Like Nikolay, the Ukrainian man who moved to western Pennsylvania, they bring their diseases with them. They don't all walk off a plane and arrive at a clinic, the way a pretty little girl named Valentina did.

At a meeting of the Northeast Tuberculosis Controllers Association in Saratoga Springs, New York, in late 1999, I sat next to Dr. Abby Greenberg, the director of disease control of the Nassau County Department of Health, just east of New York City on Long Island. She told me that an adopted Russian child with active tuberculosis had been seen at Winthrop University Hospital, a major academic center in Nassau County. It was news that I hoped I would never hear: A case of active tuberculosis in a child is bad enough, but active tuberculosis in a child from Russia raises the specter not only of TB but of multi-drug-resistant TB.

We were able to contact the family, a lovely couple; to protect their privacy we will call them Fran and Steve. After years of trying to have a baby, they had decided to adopt. Fran, an open, fast-talking dynamo with curly blonde hair, came from a Polish family and worked as an office manager. Steve, of Danish descent, was a big, quiet man, a friendly bear, 6 feet 4 inches in his stocking feet. He owned a home-improvement contracting company. Both were in their thirties.

Fran and Steve had learned that it was relatively easy to adopt a child from Russia, and they had found an agency that specialized in Russian adoptions. Americans adopt more than 120,000 children every year, both domestically and abroad.[27] The legal process in Russia would not take too long, once the planning and paperwork had been completed, which was important because they couldn't take months off from work. As an office manager, Fran felt she could handle the mountains of paperwork the adoption required. It would be expensive. Their fees and expenses could be expected to amount to about $20,000.

Fran and Steve lived in a suburban town on Long Island, New York. They could give their baby a healthy childhood in a comfortable home with grass and trees and other kids to play with, in a good school district, with lots of friends and family nearby. Good medical care was around the corner, if needed; a medical school and several university hospitals were within driving distance.

The adoption agency told them that a baby girl was available from an orphanage in a city in the far east of Russia. The baby's mother had given her up at birth. Fran and Steve received a 5-minute videotape of baby Valentina, who was then nearly a year old. They asked Dr. Jane Aronson, a well-known specialist in infectious diseases of children at Winthrop University Hospital, to review the tape. Dr. Aronson has evaluated more than 800 children adopted from abroad. She looked at the videotape, which showed the baby naked, sitting up in her crib and moving about. From all appearances, the baby seemed normal.

Go for it! they decided. In late October of 1999, Fran and Steve flew overnight on Finnair from Kennedy Airport in New York to Helsinki, then changed for a 2-hour flight to Sheremetevo, Moscow's international airport. It was a dark place, with disorderly crowds trying to push through the inordinate wait for immigration, passport control, and customs. They expected to rest in Moscow for a day to adjust to the 8-hour time difference from New York.

Instead, representatives of the adoption agency immediately picked them up and drove them miles through Moscow's sprawling suburbs, past farms, junkyards, and spanking new 25-story condos. A gray, smelly, cough-producing smog hung over the city, the product of heavy traffic and ancient Soviet cars. Finally they reached the airport for domestic flights.

All passengers, whether foreigners or Russians, had to show passports. Russia has an internal passport system, and Russians who travel within the country have passports that are more thumbed and stamped than those of most Western business people. After the passport checks and the luggage inspections, Fran and Steve went to the departure lounge, a dingy, cramped room overlooking the airfield. From there they were herded down some dark stairs and clambered into an ancient crowded bus with no seats, which took them across the tarmac to the plane. At the bottom of the stairs leading up to the plane, a chunky woman in an airline uniform checked their flight tickets, their boarding passes, and their passports yet again.

"Everybody on the plane was drunk," Steve recalled. "Each row had its own bottle of vodka. There was a long line for the toilets. Finally I realized they were going there to smoke. The back of the airplane smelled like a nicotine factory. The toilets smelled terrible, and there was no water to wash your hands." Exhausted and culture-shocked, Fran and Steve finally reached their destination, a shabby industrial city. Beggars approached them on the street, knowing that they were Americans.

Their hotel was clean but had no heat. In fact, the entire city had no heat. Like many Russian cities, it was heated by a central steam plant. Steam courses through huge pipes along the streets and over the roads, but if the central plant breaks down, nobody has heat.

It was cold in the hotel and in the orphanage. To Fran, the orphanage looked like a run-down, two-story suburban school. "The children were brought to a kind of family room as if they were being showcased," she said. Only about 14 of the approximately 90 children in the orphanage were up for adoption; the rest had been left there temporarily because their parents couldn't take care of them. The children in the orphanage were in two age groups: under about 4, and from 4 to about 11. After that age, they were moved to an orphanage for older children. And at about the age of 16, they were on their own.

Two women took care of about 16 children, dressing them, bathing them, feeding them. They worked fast. "They fed six kids while I was still feeding Valentina," Fran recalled. The Russian attendants were doing the best they could. Valentina slept in a room crowded with 20 or 30 cribs. The children didn't wear diapers because there weren't any. When they soiled their clothes overnight, "they slept in doodie," Fran said. They got clean clothes in the morning. Before they were a year old, they were taught to sit on ordinary pails to have a bowel movement. They were bathed in cold water because there wasn't any hot water. Fran brought disposable diapers for Valentina.

Fran and Steve learned little about Valentina's medical history. Her mother was 26 and had given birth to Valentina a month prematurely, while she was on the way to the hospital. She had not received any prenatal care. This was her fifth pregnancy, but only her third surviving child. Valentina's two siblings lived in far eastern Russia, and she would probably never meet them. They learned nothing about the father.

Valentina had weighed only 5 pounds at birth. She had spent 3 months in the hospital before she was sent to the orphanage. The orphanage people told Fran and Steve that she had been very sick with pneumonia and bronchitis, and had been in and out of the hospital several times. Fran said, "All the kids get sick in the orphanage there. They were sneezing and coughing." Valentina did not look as good in person as she had in the videotape. She was thin and had a rash on her face. Although she was small, she was the biggest of the children being adopted. At 13 months, Valentina weighed just 14 pounds and had not yet started teething. My colleague Dr. George McSherry, a pediatrician who evaluates many children adopted from abroad, tells me that an American child that age usually weighs around 21 pounds, and that most children have at least a few teeth by then. Of course, she had been born prematurely, which perhaps explained some of the lag.

As soon as Fran and Steve got home to Long Island in early November 1999, they took Valentina to Aronson for a checkup. They saw her on a Wednesday. Valentina's skin test for tuberculosis was positive, but that might have been because almost all Russian children get BCG vaccination. Nevertheless, Aronson ordered a chest X-ray and sent Fran and Steve home with Valentina. The moment they walked in the door, the telephone rang. Dr. Aronson wanted them to bring Valentina to the hospital on Friday morning at 6 A.M. for a CAT scan. There was something suspicious on her chest X-ray.

The CAT scan showed that Valentina had active tuberculosis affecting the upper lobe of her right lung and also some nearby lymph nodes. Aronson and her colleague Dr. Philip Lee decided to admit Valentina to the hospital.

If Valentina had been an adult, the doctors would most likely have had her cough up some sputum to see if it contained tuberculosis bacteria. But Valentina was hardly more than a baby, and infants don't have the strength to cough up sputum. Instead, they swallow it. The only way doctors can get a sputum sample from a baby is from the stomach. Valentina stayed in the hospital for 3 days. Each morning before breakfast, a thin nasogastric tube was threaded down from her nose into her stomach. Through the tube, doctors suctioned up sputum that she had swallowed overnight. Valentina cried throughout the uncomfortable procedure.

The doctors also performed a spinal tap, inserting a thin needle between the bones of Valentina's spine and withdrawing fluid from around the spinal cord. When infants and young children have tuberculosis, they may develop a common, often devastating, complication, meningitis, in which tuberculosis infects the tissues around the brain and spinal cord. Valentina's doctors needed to know whether there were TB bacteria in her spinal fluid.

"They told us that the quick tests [the sputum smear and the spinal tap] were negative, and they gave us all these medications," Fran said. The doctors sent the sputum to the Centers for Disease Control and Prevention in Atlanta to be cultured. It would take weeks. Once the bacteria had grown in the cultures, they would be tested for drug sensitivity to make sure that Valentina was getting the right medications. Since Valentina came from Russia, there was a possibility that she had been infected with multi-drug-resistant tuberculosis, which would make treatment far more difficult. Meanwhile, Valentina had to take the medications that were most likely to be effective against her tuberculosis. She was given a drug cocktail called RIPE (rifampin, isoniazid, pyrazinamide, and ethambutol).

Fran and Steve were devastated. "We waited 6 months to adopt her," Fran said, "and now this news!" Like most babies with active TB, at least she wasn't contagious. Since Valentina was too young to cough out the bugs, she couldn't infect Fran, Steve, their family members, or her playmates.

They sought second opinions from a lung specialist and an infectious diseases expert at the State University of New York at Stony Brook, near their home. These experts confirmed the diagnosis. Valentina had active tuberculosis and needed to be treated.

Perhaps just as worrying as Valentina's TB, it was very likely that some of the other children in the orphanage were also infected by the same strain of TB, since all the children had probably been exposed at the same time to the same bacteria that infected Valentina. When Fran and Steve were adopting Valentina, another American couple and a single American woman were there to adopt other children. No one knows whether those children got the same careful medical attention that Valentina got when they got to the United States. Do these children, too, now have active tuberculosis? Do they have latent TB infection, at risk of progressing to active tuberculosis?

Every day, Fran and Steve gave Valentina the four medicines they hoped would cure her. At the beginning they had problems, but they worked out a way around them. Isoniazid, a liquid, went into Valentina's juice. The pills, ethambutol, pyrazinamide, and rifampin, were crushed and put into the fruit puree she ate after dinner. The medicines made her irritable and gave her diarrhea. She got a rash.

People from the Suffolk County Department of Health, informed as required by law of a reported case of tuberculosis, said that they had to come and see that Valentina got directly observed therapy (DOT). Steve explained to them that Valentina received some medication during the day in her juice. The other medications she got after dinner in her pureed fruit. "We eat at about 6. Then she goes to bed. Have someone come over around 6," he said. The health department worker said they worked from 9 to 5. "After that, we never heard from them," Steve said. Fran and Steve continued giving Valentina her medications on their own, effective schedule.

Valentina began to blossom. She was a pretty child with dark hazel eyes and light brown hair. She gained 5 pounds in less than 4 months. She grew taller. Before Christmas, she learned to walk. By February 2000, she had eight teeth. By the summertime, she was delighting her parents with her enthusiasm during their visits to the beach.

"At first, she missed the orphanage and all the other children," Fran said. "Now she laughs all day. She's a happy child, a survivor. She's inquisitive. In the orphanage she was not alive. She lacked love. There are days when she just wants to be hugged all day. She's very attached to Steve. When he comes home, she's thrilled. She's brought so much joy into our lives that we can't imagine life without her."

After Valentina had been taking her medicines for over 3 months, the CDC reported that the cultures of the three sputum samples retrieved from her stomach by the nasogastric tube were negative. They were unable to grow any bacteria from them. But this wasn't surprising. Negative cultures in a case of active TB are not that uncommon, particularly in a child. It's difficult to retrieve sputum from the stomach, and the stomach acids might have killed the TB bacteria.

Because the cultures were negative, there was no way of knowing for sure if the antibiotics Valentina was taking would cure her TB. Since she is now growing well, however, we can be pretty sure that the standard drugs her doctors chose were the right drugs to cure her. By 2001, she had religiously completed her course of medications, carefully watched over by her doting parents. She will always test positive on a skin test, but she is highly likely to have a long, healthy life, is highly unlikely to relapse with TB, and needs absolutely no medical follow-up.

We don't know and probably never will know where Valentina's TB came from. Since TB infection usually requires prolonged contact, it was very unlikely that she got it from her mother, who had abandoned her at birth. Valentina and her mother had not had any contact after birth. It's possible, but very rare, for tuberculosis to be transmitted through the placental blood from mother to child. Most likely Valentina was infected by a caregiver at the orphanage, a health-care worker at the hospital where she stayed before she got to the orphanage, or someone who visited the orphanage often, such as a relative or parent of one of the other children. Perhaps one of those people had had contact with a former prisoner or someone employed at a prison as a housekeeper, secretary, or guard who came home every night to eat and sleep with his or her family. Most Russian prisons lack even the simplest infection control procedures.

Valentina's story raises a much bigger and more painful problem: How many of the 16,000 or more children who are adopted from abroad each year like Valentina are never correctly investigated and appropriately treated, as she was by Dr Aronson?

I shudder to speculate, but an experience just a few years ago suggests that the answer may not be encouraging.

In 1998, as described in Chapter 6, "Inside the Gulag," I visited Tomsk in Siberia and saw the disastrous TB problem in a typical Siberian oblast, or region, for the first time. When I came back to Moscow, I was interviewed for National Public Radio's *Morning Edition* by NPR reporter Anne Garrells and was asked to give a thorough, accurate account of the TB situation in Russia. She was one of the very first to call attention to Russia's serious and growing tuberculosis problem. As part of her report, she gave the New Jersey Medical School National Tuberculosis Center's national TB information line, 1-800-4TB-DOCS, for listeners to call for information about TB.

By the end of the week in which the report was broadcast, I had had three calls, all giving the same scenario: The caller had adopted a child from Russia or another country of the former Soviet Union, the child had a positive tuberculin skin test (which means that the child very likely has a latent TB infection) and therefore a 1 in 10 risk of developing active tuberculosis during its lifetime, and the local pediatrician told the mother not to worry about the positive skin test "because all children in Russia get BCG vaccination," and so no further tests were ever done. It wasn't just small-town pediatricians who gave out this erroneous information. One mother who persisted and took her child to an infectious diseases specialist at the state university medical center got the same message. Furthermore, she said, friends of hers who had adopted children from areas of the Far East that are hotbeds of TB had never had their children tested for TB. Neither the doctors nor the parents had thought of it.

Although the positive skin test in children adopted from TB hot spots might be due to vaccination, one cannot really tell. BCG is not effective in preventing tuberculosis later in life, so at least some cases of latent TB infection and very likely some easily preventable and treatable cases of *active* tuberculosis are being missed in these adopted children.

I hope that if the child develops symptoms of tuberculosis—failure to thrive, weakness, cough, fever, and chills—the physician will think of TB, diagnose it, and treat it before irreparable damage is done. I also hope that if the child develops active tuberculosis later in life, it will not be the multi-drug-resistant form from the former Soviet Union or other hot spots that is not only so difficult to treat, but that spreads as easily as ordinary tuberculosis. For the safety of the rest of us in the world to which TB can spread through the air, I hope this child's infection will be ordinary TB, sensitive to the old-fashioned drugs we have had in our arsenal for 30, 40, and 50 years —because we don't have any new ones.

5

Smoke and Mirrors in Moscow

Enter Alex Goldfarb

I first made contact with Dr. Alex Goldfarb on a conference call from Moscow in May 1997. I was in the utilitarian offices of the Public Health Research Institute on First Avenue in New York, a plain white brick building across the street from Bellevue Hospital, where I trained as a medical student, intern, and resident in the 1960s. Goldfarb was on his cell phone from Moscow. He is seldom separated from it. He probably takes it into the shower.

Goldfarb was a friend of George Soros, the billionaire international philanthropist and financier. Several years earlier, Goldfarb had helped Soros in a majestic, unpublicized, and now forgotten $100 million campaign to "save the Russian scientists" from defecting to terrorist nations after the Soviet Union fell apart in 1991. Now Goldfarb was asking me to help with his current mission, a Soros-funded effort by the Public Health Research Institute, Goldfarb's employer, to deal with the epidemic of multi-drug-resistant tuberculosis in Russia. Goldfarb was the first person to call Soros's attention to the problem of tuberculosis in Russia. Before Soros got involved, there was virtually zero donor money going into any Russian antituberculosis program, and their TB cases were rising at a frightening rate.

Who was Goldfarb, and how in the world did he and, through him, Soros get involved? It is a fascinating and tangled story of family, politics, and science.

During World War II, when Russia was an important ally of the United States, Goldfarb's maternal grandfather, Gregory Heifets, ran the Soviet intelligence operation in San Francisco. Heifets returned to Moscow in 1944.

Because of his stature and experience as a high-ranking member of the establishment, Joseph Stalin immediately got him involved in his plan to establish a Soviet Socialist Jewish republic in the Crimea, in southern Russia on the Black Sea, and thereby get Jewish investment from abroad. Heifets, who was Jewish but not Orthodox or even particularly religious, was a key person in plans for the new republic. After Israel was founded in 1947, however, Stalin abruptly changed his mind and abandoned the whole project. He rewarded all the people involved, including Heifets, by putting them in prison.

After Stalin's death in 1953, Goldfarb's grandfather was released. Goldfarb was 6 or 7 years old at the time. "I remember him as an old, wrinkled man who didn't talk too much," he said. "Perhaps to keep himself occupied, he started to teach me English. He had lived most of his life in Europe and the United States. He was very cosmopolitan. He spoke several languages. Even though he had been jailed by Stalin, he remained a loyal Communist."

The family was privileged by Soviet standards, but not rich. "I grew up in a big, old-fashioned apartment in downtown Moscow, right next to the Bolshoi theater. My grandfather's family and my family lived in the apartment. It probably had three bedrooms. It was far better than anybody else around us had," Goldfarb recalled. It was common at the time for entire multigenerational Soviet families to live in a single room and share kitchens and bathrooms with their neighbors.

Alex Goldfarb's father, David Goldfarb, was a professor of microbiology at Moscow University. Alex was to follow in his footsteps. During the Khrushchev era, from 1956 to 1967, there was a thaw. Free discussions were allowed. Reforms were begun. People were released from prisons. There was a political and cultural renaissance.

In this heady atmosphere of intellectual freedom, Alex Goldfarb entered Moscow University in 1964 to study microbiology. The university was a center for free thinking and dissent. But in 1967, when Goldfarb was 20, the Soviets invaded Czechoslovakia to clamp down on the new freedoms in that country, which had gone too far. The thaw was suddenly over.

Goldfarb graduated from Moscow University in 1969 and entered graduate school to continue his studies in microbiology. Dissident groups—probably no more than 200 or 300 people all told—were stubbornly pressing for government reform and a more open society. Members of these groups gathered information about abuses and passed it on to the West through friendly foreign reporters and foreign embassy people, creating a network that has aided Goldfarb's activities to this day. Goldfarb helped organize the smuggling into Russia of banned books, such as George Orwell's *Animal Farm* and *1984* and the Bible, books that a Soviet citizen could be imprisoned for possessing.

Because he spoke such good English, Goldfarb became the spokesperson for the entire loose group of dissidents. "I was running around Moscow, arranging interviews with the *New York Times*, hosting American congressmen. Support groups in the United States and Canada helped us. A Canadian family I had never met sent me $60 a month. With that money and what I earned by tutoring, I had almost enough to live on," he said.

During this time, Goldfarb spent a couple of years acting as the informal assistant and secretary to Andrei Sakharov, who was a key figure among the dissidents. Sakharov was a Russian nuclear scientist who became an internationally recognized spokesperson for human rights, and consequently was sent into internal exile in Russia. He won the Nobel Peace Prize in 1975.

All the while he was engaged in his dissident activities, Goldfarb was in graduate school, working in molecular genetics. The institute where he was studying was part of the Soviet atomic energy establishment. Goldfarb came to realize that the further he advanced with his studies, the more valuable he would become to the Soviet establishment and the more difficult it would be for him to leave the Soviet Union. He might be trapped for the rest of his life.

In 1973, when he was 26, Goldfarb dropped out of graduate school just short of his Ph.D. and applied for an exit visa. At that time, exit visas were allowed for people who had ethnic connections to another land, as Goldfarb had to Israel, since the Soviet Union classified him as a Jew. It was the only way out to freedom. "My family was worried. A couple of my friends had ended up in jail. The visa was denied." Stubborn as ever, Goldfarb persisted in his dissident activities and his contacts with Westerners and journalists.

But when a dissident became too effective, he was either thrown in jail or thrown out of the country. In 1975, Goldfarb was suddenly called into the section of the Ministry of the Interior in charge of passports. A bureaucrat told him, "We have changed our minds. You can go. You must write a paper saying that you have renounced Soviet citizenship. You will be an ex-citizen. You can leave." Goldfarb would become stateless. They gave him 2 weeks to get out.

The Molecular Biologist

After his hurried departure, Goldfarb got his Ph.D. from the Weizmann Institute in Israel, then landed a postdoctoral appointment at the Max Planck Institute in Munich, Germany.

From early in his scientific career, Goldfarb had been working on understanding the way antibiotic drug resistance occurs. His special interest was RNA transcription, the process by which genetic information is picked up from the central DNA in every cell and then expressed in the cell. Transcription is carried out by an enzyme called RNA polymerase. DNA, which comprises the genetic code, issues the order; RNA carries it out.

Goldfarb was particularly interested in how RNA polymerase was the target of rifampin, then a new and exciting drug, and to this day our most important and powerful drug against TB. Once rifampin gets inside the tuberculosis-infected cell, it blocks transcription, the message from DNA to RNA, in the TB bacteria. The disabled bacteria die. Rifampin kills TB bacteria, but it doesn't harm ordinary human cells. Goldfarb discovered that when rifampin didn't work, it was because a mutation in the RNA polymerase of the TB bacteria had made the bacteria resistant to the antibiotic. Such information is important for scientists who are trying to develop better drugs to treat tuberculosis, because it gives them clues about where to target a new drug.

Goldfarb's professor at the Max Planck Institute recommended him to Columbia University in New York, where he soon moved. Goldfarb's skills and knowledge quickly attracted impressive research grants from the National Institutes of Health. He then spent 10 productive years at Columbia. However, the stubborn nature, disregard for authority, and independent ways that had served him so well as a dissident—but which are anathema in academic circles— got him into a dispute with the temporary head of his department. In the ultimate academic rejection, Goldfarb was denied tenure at the university. In academic circles, that is akin to being declared stateless and thrown out of the Soviet Union.

Besides effectively ending his career at Columbia, Goldfarb's failure to gain tenure tainted him in the eyes of other universities and medical research centers. This happened despite his strong record of scientific achievement and the fact that when he left Columbia, he had two grants from the National Institutes of Health worth half a million dollars a year, grants that would pay research staff and buy laboratory equipment and supplies, as well as provide a hefty percentage for a sponsoring university.

Ultimately, in 1992, Goldfarb found a home with the Public Health Research Institute, a New York City institution founded in 1941 by the legendary Mayor Fiorello LaGuardia. This independent institute (PHRI, as it is universally known) lives only on its grants from the National Institutes of

Health, the National Science Foundation, and other agencies—grants that are given because of the quality of research. Unlike most other research centers, PHRI has no endowment or support from government, nor is it a part of any university—it has its own governance structure, and thus its independence. Perhaps the independence of PHRI was a better match for Goldfarb's iconoclastic personality, as they have been collaborating effectively since he joined the staff in 1992.

Billionaire Seeks Dissident

In 1987, before he had joined the PHRI, Goldfarb had had his "15 minutes of fame," and this had brought him to the attention of Soros. Goldfarb's family had remained in Moscow when he left, and his father, the retired microbiology professor, became a personal friend of an American journalist, Nicholas Daniloff of *US News and World Report*. Daniloff was arrested in Moscow as a U.S. spy, in retaliation for the FBI's arrest of a Russian spy in New York. The Russians began building a case against David Goldfarb as well.

In the fall of 1987, U.S. President Ronald Reagan and Soviet President Mikhail Gorbachev held a summit meeting in Reykjavik, Iceland. Alex Goldfarb flew to Iceland and demonstrated with a poster outside the hall where the summit was taking place. "Let my father go," he pleaded.

It worked. About a month later the Russian spy arrested in New York was exchanged for the American journalist Daniloff, and David Goldfarb was part of the package. Both he and Alex's mother were flown out of Russia. The story was front-page news, hailed as a sign that Gorbachev was serious about perestroika, the "restructuring" of the Soviet state. But this front page news brought Goldfarb and his father to the attention of George Soros.

Days after the rescue of his father, Alex Goldfarb remembers, "Somebody called me, probably from Human Rights Watch, an activist group supported in part by George Soros, and said, 'Mr. Soros wants to meet you and your father.' Until then I had only thought of Soros as a rich guy who was interested in good causes. The meeting was supposed to take place on a day when there was a huge New York snowstorm. My father was sitting in a hospital bed in Columbia-Presbyterian Medical Center. He was a diabetic, and he had gangrene affecting his foot, and lung cancer as well. We waited for Mr. Soros's visit. Finally I gave up and left. Then George Soros, the billionaire, actually came to see my father in the hospital.

"My father couldn't have cared less. As far as he was concerned, Soros was just another American. They talked about politics, but that was really my department. My father was involved in managing his ailments."

Soon afterward, Soros got in touch with Goldfarb again and invited him to a meeting in his Fifth Avenue apartment. "It was a typical rich man's apartment, two floors overlooking Central Park. Huge. It had marble and paintings, and it was well furnished." Soros explained that he wanted to set up a private foundation in Russia, as he had done in Poland and China. He wanted to promote a democratic way of life, what he called an "open society." Goldfarb was highly skeptical. He said that the money would be stolen or taken over by the KGB. Nevertheless, for the next 5 years, Goldfarb was invited to occasional meetings with Soros at social gatherings that involved an entourage of antiestablishment types, usually made up of assorted Russian expatriates, about five or six people, some more and some less famous.

"One day in 1992, around Thanksgiving, one of Soros's people called me. I was in bad shape. My father had died the year before. I'd been kicked out of Columbia. I was divorced, with child support to pay. I had no money. I was living in Queens (a middle-class but unfashionable area of New York City). I had just started at PHRI," Goldfarb said. He was invited to a meeting at the National Academy of Sciences in Washington, a meeting with a special purpose.

Soros wanted to make a major grant to save and support the academic community in the former Soviet Union, to help Russian scientists whose expertise and knowledge were being lost. The scientists weren't being paid. They saw greener pastures in terrorist countries. Soros hoped to keep the scientists at work on serious science in Russia. Russian President Boris Yeltsin had just introduced "shock therapy," and most Russians had lost all their savings. International economists called it "meltdown." Unemployment was rampant, many people weren't getting paid, life expectancy was dropping, and people were begging in the Metro and on the streets. Soros asked Goldfarb to run the Russian science project.

Saving Russian Scientists

In deciding to put Goldfarb in charge, Soros made a good choice. In his early forties, Goldfarb was a respected international scientist. He was also a brilliant politician. He is husky, vigorous, unconventional, and so fast in his thinking that many people can't keep up with him. Though some people —especially some bureaucrats—are threatened by his stubborn manner, good connections, and obvious successes, he is also friendly and likable, with wavy, dark hair only tinged with gray, a scruffy beard, and the deep hazel-brown eyes that so many Russians have. You can see why women find him attractive.

Soros trusted Goldfarb. Goldfarb certainly knew Russia. He knew Russian scientists, because he had started out as one of them. He knew influential people, because he'd either gone to school with them or had contact with them in his dissident days. He knew how to administer million dollar programs because of his research grants.

Soros set up the International Science Foundation in Russia, with headquarters in Moscow, and gave Goldfarb the task of distributing $100 million. The foundation gave grants and stipends to scientists in all fields to keep them and the system functioning. Goldfarb cut back his laboratory work at the Public Health Research Institute to half time and began commuting to Moscow. With a staff of about 100, Goldfarb selected the appropriate scientists and distributed the money in a careful and controlled manner. Soros pushed him to spend the money as fast as possible, so that it would have the most impact. With the ruble crashing and the economy collapsing, $100 million had the impact of $10 billion at that time, but in 2 years it would be worth much less.

The management office that dealt with finance for the International Science Foundation was located at the Public Health Research Institute. "There were no banks in Russia," Goldfarb explained. "No one had computers. There were no laws, no Federal Deposit Insurance Corporation. Russians still don't have personal checking accounts. It was a wild situation that reminded me of E. L. Doctorow's *Ragtime*." He insists that "not a penny was stolen from our operation."

Working with Goldfarb in Moscow was Dr. Oksana I. Ponomarenko, a smart biologist whose connections in the Moscow hierarchy were almost as good as his. She has a talent for administration and diplomacy and, like Goldfarb, is seldom separated from her cell phone. Between Goldfarb and Ponomarenko, in 3 1/2 years, the International Science Foundation efficiently and quietly distributed $100 million of Soros's money and almost single-handedly saved the Russian scientific community. Of course, the effort was noticed by Russian scientists and the politicians in the ministries concerned with health and science.

By 1996, after the International Science Foundation had distributed all $100 million of Soros's money to Russian scientists and closed down, Goldfarb was able to return full time to his work on antibiotic resistance, working in collaboration with colleagues in Moscow and also in contact with long-time friends and researchers in antibiotic resistance in New York, such as Alex Tomasz and Nobel laureate Joshua Lederberg of Rockefeller University, both friends of Soros. They were concerned that the overuse and misuse of antibiotics in raising livestock and in treating trivial infections was making more bugs impervious to antibiotics. It wasn't just TB. Almost-incurable infections of several kinds, often acquired in the hospital by desperately ill patients, were on the rise.

Beginning the Battle with Russian TB

The reason I was taking part in that conference call with Goldfarb in May 1997 was that earlier in the year, Goldfarb had visited Soros in London and convinced him that antibiotic drug resistance and tuberculosis were major problems in Russia. Soros promised to contribute $3 million to support laboratories to monitor the problems. The Public Health Research Institute would supervise the program. Russia would get two sophisticated labs: one for a modern tuberculosis control program, and another to investigate antibiotic-resistant hospital infections. Each lab would cost $1.5 million to build and would be based at an existing institution. The TB lab—which is what I got involved in—was to be a world-class laboratory in Moscow that would be a reference lab to check the results of regional labs in Russia.

The Russian Ministry of Health had told Goldfarb and Soros that the country's leading TB expert was Dr. Alexey A. Priymak, phthisiologist in chief of Russia and head of the "Priymak institute" at the Dostoyevsky Hospital in Moscow, one of Russia's leading TB centers. Since Goldfarb had not yet entered the world of global TB politics, particularly as far as Russia was concerned, he agreed with the Ministry of Health's recommendation that the TB lab be built at the Priymak institute, and Soros went along. With major fanfare, the Soros gift and project were announced at a joint press conference in Moscow with Soros, Goldfarb, and the Russian minister of health, Tatyana Dmitriyeva, in late June 1997.

Although a "done deal," to give the project legitimacy, Goldfarb needed to assemble a committee of experts to evaluate Priymak's lab in Moscow before the Soros-funded upgrade could begin. He asked me to get involved. However, I expressed my reservations to Lew Weinstein, the president of the Public Health Research Institute, explaining that Priymak was not respected in the international TB community. In fact, he was a virtual pariah because of his archaic views. The World Health Organization and the U.S. Centers for Disease Control and Prevention were so concerned about his influence as Russia's top TB doctor that the CDC had funded an extensive study tour for about ten people on Priymak's top staff, to visit major TB public health and academic centers in the United States. As part of this tour, they had visited my TB center, a few months before that first conference call with Goldfarb.

When Priymak and his team visited the New Jersey Medical School National Tuberculosis Center in Newark, they spent a whole day observing our evidence-based results. About 98 percent of our patients were being cured, even though many of them lived in deprived circumstances, were unemployed, or were homeless. We almost never needed to do surgery. We seldom needed to hospitalize patients. We treated patients discreetly, on an ambulatory basis, at home or on the job, while they got on with their lives. We thought these were exceptional results, but Priymak was totally (although cordially) dismissive of our and the WHO's directly observed therapy (DOTS) strategy, however successful it was. "DOTS is for Africa, not Russia," Priymak said, as he and his colleagues left our TB center at the end of the day.

I gave Lew Weinstein my opinion of Priymak, and he had already heard the opinions of the WHO and the CDC. I explained my serious reservations about Priymak's operation in Russia, Weinstein assured me that the evaluation committee was not to be a rubber stamp, but was to give a fair, honest assessment of Priymak's laboratory.

I finally met Alex Goldfarb in person early in the morning on Wednesday, July 9, 1997, when I arrived in Moscow to evaluate Priymak's lab at the Dostoyevsky Hospital. With me were two TB lab experts, Dr. Max Salfinger, a physician who heads the Wadsworth Reference Laboratory of the New York State Department of Health in Albany, and Yvonne Hale, biological administrator at the Bureau of Laboratories at the Florida State Department of Health. Little did we know that our trip would turn into a strange, smoke-and-mirrors, cloak-and-dagger adventure with the feel of a John LeCarré novel about the Cold War and the Evil Empire.

The old Dostoyevsky Hospital, where the Priymak institute is situated, is a glorious building in the Russian classical style, painted goldenrod yellow and white, with a stone statue of the great novelist Fyodor Dostoyevsky in the front garden. This graceful structure was built at the beginning of the nineteenth century as a school for daughters of the nobility, served as a hospital for Napoleon's wounded soldiers when the French emperor made the mistake of invading Russia, and has been a TB hospital for many years. Dostoyevsky was born nearby and died of tuberculosis—hence the name.

The hospital's long, echoing corridors, marble staircases, high ceilings, and domed rooms are now run down. Built before electricity and central heating, the building has had the blessing and the curse of being landmarked.

Even if the money were to become available, it would be extremely difficult to get permission to make the alterations necessary to create modern
laboratories, modern patient rooms, modern operating rooms, and computerized systems.

Beyond the physical condition of the building, we were appalled by
what we saw. Patients underwent serious surgery for TB, something that
almost never happened in other industrialized countries. They lived in the
hospital for a year or more, in drab, high-ceilinged rooms divided by parti-
tions. The rooms were more like dormitories than like hospital rooms as we
think of them. Many difficult cases of TB were referred to the hospital from
across Russia. About 80 percent of these patients had drug-resistant and
exotic forms of the disease. The hospital even had a ward for patients with
TB of the eye!

Salfinger and I saw a young girl of 16 who had been flown across Russia's
nine time zones from Vladivostok, a port in the far eastern region of Russia
on the Pacific Ocean, to undergo drastic surgery to remove parts of both
her lungs at the Priymak institute. When Salfinger and I saw her after surgery,
she had drainage tubes protruding from surgical wounds on both sides of
her chest. We were stunned. Neither of us could remember ever having seen
major surgery to remove parts of both lungs at the same time.

Back home in New Jersey, I would have treated such a young woman
with drugs to which her TB was sensitive for 6 months or so. She would
probably never have been hospitalized and almost certainly would not have
needed surgery. She would have taken her medication on an outpatient
basis; it would have been delivered to her home or school by an outreach
worker who would have watched her take the pills. In less than a month,
she would have begun to feel better, but the outreach worker would have
made sure that she completed the drug regimen. This is the treatment protocol we call DOT. With careful outpatient follow-up, this patient would
have done well and continued to go to school with minimal disruption of
her life.

Salfinger and I spoke to the doctors at the Priymak institute about the
drugs they prescribed for TB patients, and found that they didn't follow the
World Health Organization protocol that is endorsed by 128 countries.
Tuberculosis bacteria mutate easily, and patients with active tuberculosis
carry hundreds of millions of organisms; thus the TB patient must be always
be initially treated with at least four drugs at the same time. The first kills
most of the TB bacteria, the second drug kills the bacteria that are or become
resistant to the first drug, the third drug kills those that are resistant to the
first two drugs, and so on. Four drugs are used because some of the patient's

TB bacteria may already be resistant to one or more antibiotics at the beginning of treatment. TB experts around the world agree that failure to administer enough potent drugs against tuberculosis simultaneously for the right length of time invariably leads to drug resistance. And if the patient is contagious (as most patients with TB of the lung are, especially if they are not receiving proper therapy), that resistance is contagious.

Not only did the Priymak institute not subscribe to the standard four-drug regimen of isoniazid, rifampin, pyrazinamide, and ethambutol, it had been an extremely outspoken opponent of it. Four of the leading organizations in the global fight against TB—the World Health Organization, the U.S. Centers for Disease Control and Prevention, the International Union against Tuberculosis and Lung Disease, and the Royal Netherlands Tuberculosis Association (KNCV, from its initials in Dutch)—had been worried about TB in Russia for years. They regarded the Priymak institute as a center of unorthodox ideas and ineffective TB treatment and an outspoken opponent of the World Health Organization's comprehensive strategy to control TB, DOTS. (DOTS, which originally stood for "directly observed therapy short course," a specific menu of elements related to TB control, has come to be regarded as the WHO trademark for good TB control.) So it should have come as no surprise, when we got to Moscow and visited the Priymak institute, to find that instead of following the proven DOTS regimen, doctors at the institute were treating patients with their own creative cocktails of drugs. One doctor didn't like to use the powerful and proven rifampin at all because she thought it had too many side effects. Other doctors liked to add drugs or vitamins that they thought would help the patients, although they could not cite any studies to show that the treatment worked. We knew that experimenting willy-nilly with drugs in this way, instead of sticking with a proven, effective regimen of multiple drugs given together, was inevitably encouraging the development of multi-drug-resistant tuberculosis.

Nevertheless, despite what we and international TB leaders thought of Priymak's way of treating patients, our mission was to evaluate his laboratories.

More Bad News

Our first exposure to the unorthodox practices of the Priymak institute, Wednesday afternoon July 9, had been a depressing day for the three of us. We agreed that the global TB establishment was quite correct in its criticism of Priymak's policies and procedures. The problem was that Soros, Goldfarb, and PHRI had already publicly committed their support and prestige to this undeserving group. We were jet-lagged and tired. I suggested that we invite my old TB colleague, Professor Alexander Khomenko, to dinner at our hotel that evening. I knew Khomenko from many international meetings and from the International Union against Tuberculosis and Lung Disease, where we had both served on the executive committee. Khomenko had also worked on TB at the World Health Organization in Geneva some years previously. He was a professor and an academician of the Russian Academy of Sciences and formerly of the Academy of Sciences of the Soviet Union, the highest distinction a scientist can achieve in Russia.

Khomenko was 14 when Hitler invaded Russia in 1941. In those desperate times, he was drafted into working as a nurse in a hospital and then as a military feldsher, sort of a physician's assistant. He did so well that when the war ended he was sent to train as a doctor. As he was finishing his studies, he became ill with tuberculosis, but he managed to continue his education. He had severe pleuritis, a painful tuberculosis infection of the membranes around the lungs and inside the chest. He had a hemorrhage from the lungs. "It was a terrible time, with starvation and privation," according to his wife, Dr. Nina Khomenko, who married him when they were both medical students. Khomenko probably would have died except that Nina Khomenko's father, a high-ranking official, managed to get streptomycin, then the new miracle antibiotic against tuberculosis, from Soviet troops who had brought it with them when they were returning from Germany. Alexander Khomenko was treated with the old method, pneumothorax, and with the new streptomycin. Within a year and a half, with treatment and good food, he recovered. From then on, he had a brilliant career dedicated to stopping tuberculosis.

Khomenko had had some rough times when the Soviet Union came apart in 1991. Mikhail Gorbachev, the head of the Soviet Union, was challenged by Boris Yeltsin, the head of Russia, the largest state within the Soviet Union. It was as if Texas had challenged the United States and managed to break up the nation. Previously there had been Soviet Union organizations and academies and other organizations and academies in the larger states, such as Russia. As fast as he could, Yeltsin abolished or downgraded the Soviet-level academies and kept and enhanced the Russian ones. It was as if the Texas Academy of Sciences were to replace the National Academy of Sciences. Khomenko for years, had been the top Soviet TB authority. He had trained most of the people in the discipline. He edited the major Soviet scientific journal on TB. Even in the current disordered state of affairs, there was no denying that he was Russia's most important TB scientist with national—and one of the few with international—credentials.

Khomenko spoke English well, and so did many members of his staff. English is the language of science. Any major player in international science must be able to read English, because most of the literature appears in English. It may take 2 or 3 years before an important research paper gets translated even into the major European languages, such as French, German, or Spanish. Scientists who speak only Russian will learn only what Russian scientists and writers have to say about TB, which most international experts regard as at least 50 years out of date.

I was looking forward to seeing my old friend again for dinner. Salfinger, Hale, and I were staying at the President Hotel, in the southern part of Moscow, across the river from the Kremlin. On Wednesday evening, as we were waiting for Khomenko, the hotel refused to let him in. I began to feel that there was something strange going on. Why were security people keeping out one of Russia's highest-ranking scientists? I went out, found him outside the hotel gate, and brought him in from the street, where he had been made to wait.

We had a pleasant dinner, and he invited us to come to see his own institute 2 days later, a Friday. He ran the Central Tuberculosis Research Institute of the Russian Academy of Medical Sciences (called the Khomenko institute to this day), a group of buildings on the leafy outskirts of Moscow near a nature preserve. But before we could visit Khomenko's institute, we would have the next day, Thursday, to complete our already planned visit to Priymak's, a task none of us was looking forward to.

On Thursday morning, the three of us returned to the Priymak institute at Dostoyevsky Hospital to see the labs we would be evaluating. Once again, we were appalled. Laboratory personnel were working with dangerous TB bacteria with no precautions. They were carrying infectious sputum in trays of open brown bottles. If someone had dropped a tray, highly infectious TB bacteria would have flown through the air.

They were spinning test tubes of TB bacteria inside a centrifuge, a standard method used to concentrate the bacteria for study. But their ancient centrifuge couldn't spin fast enough to concentrate the bacteria, which meant that the laboratory was probably underestimating the number of infections. The tubes inside the centrifuge that contained the deadly bacteria did not have safety caps. If the lid had come off the centrifuge, a cloud of these bacteria would have been sprayed all over the lab. Not only would this endanger the lab workers, it would also contaminate all the other samples in the lab.

There were no biosafety hoods, which are needed to protect workers in labs dealing with dangerous bacteria like TB. Such hoods separate lab workers from the bacteria and filter the bacteria out of the air immediately around the workers. The lab workers were not even wearing protective, tightly sealed masks. Salfinger commented that he'd seen better safety precautions when he had recently evaluated labs in war-torn Kosovo.

When we asked to see how a lab worker did a particular test, we had a very strong suspicion that the test was staged for our benefit. The worker had probably never done it before, and she was using a sample given by a drug company representative. If the test were done regularly, the lab would have to have a large supply of the chemical, not just a sample. When we asked about a mask, she pulled out a useless thin cotton one, not the specially fitted protective kind that should always be worn when dealing with any dangerous bacteria.

Things got worse. When we asked to see more of the lab, we were told that the person who had the keys had gone home. No one knew where the keys were kept.

The whole setup reminded us of a Potemkin village, the stage-set towns that Gregory Potemkin set up to show his lover, the Empress Catherine the Great of Russia, that her people were living well, when in fact they were starving.

Escape

While we were at Priymak's lab, we asked several times about making a visit to Khomenko's lab the next day, and several times we were discouraged. We were told that it was too far away, on the outskirts of Moscow. We were reminded that it would be a Friday; people would have gone home for the weekend. Clearly no one wanted us to see Khomenko's lab.

We persisted. After we arrived at the Priymak institute on Friday, and continued our inspection, Salfinger and I finally managed to leave Hale as a sort of hostage/decoy to keep Priymak's team occupied while we sneaked off to see Khomenko's institute. The biologist Oksana Ponomarenko, Goldfarb's deputy, came along with us, although she didn't seem to see much point in the visit. Khomenko helped us in this subterfuge by sending two cars to pick us up, in case one car was intercepted.

Khomenko's lab was refreshingly different. It didn't have the most modern equipment, but it seemed to adhere to and promote modern principles. Since they were using good techniques, scientists there were much more likely to get accurate results from TB cultures than those in Priymak's lab. Another sign that Khomenko's was a modern reference lab was the very large number of samples it was evaluating from other labs. Priymak's people first said that they evaluated only 20 samples a day from other labs, then they changed the number to 60 or 70 per day. They finally said they received only 300 to 400 cultures a year to confirm cultures done in other labs.

If Priymak's was actually a reference lab for 400 or 800 other labs in Russia, as we had been told, it should surely have been getting more than a few samples a week. Khomenko's lab was evaluating thousands of samples from other labs on a regular basis. Furthermore, Khomenko's lab was part of a network of international quality control labs, constantly sending its own well-checked specimens to reference labs such as the Pasteur Institute in Paris for confirmation.

What impressed us most was how open Khomenko was with us. There was no way he could have done a smoke-and-mirrors show overnight to make things look wonderful at his lab. We were confident that we saw it as it operated every day—well run and productive. Ponomarenko also saw the difference instantly and was surprised by the contrast.

So what were we going to recommend for Soros's money, given that he and Goldfarb had so publicly promised to fund Priymak's laboratory? Obviously, that decision and that whole high-profile press conference had been a huge mistake. Since an excellent laboratory already existed in Khomenko's institute, why spend $1.5 million funding a new lab at all? I was afraid our only possible recommendation, after what we had seen, was: Don't fund the Priymak lab, but do invest to improve Khomenko's lab, which is good already. I was afraid our recommendation was going to be ignored. Soros and Goldfarb were in a difficult position: People—especially such prominent people—do not like to appear wrong in public.

A Difficult Dinner

When we got back to the President Hotel late that afternoon after seeing Khomenko's lab, we knew we were already committed to a dinner with Priymak and his deputy in Le Gastronome, an exclusive restaurant on the ground floor of one of Moscow's seven Stalin-era gothic skyscrapers. We knew that the dinner was supposed to be a happy "exit interview." We were supposed to tell Priymak that we had formally approved his lab and that "the check was in the mail," so to speak.

The instant we entered the hotel lobby, Salfinger and I called Goldfarb (who was to meet us at the restaurant) on his cell phone and told him to get over to our hotel as fast as he could. When he arrived an hour later (thanks to Moscow's terrible traffic), we grabbed him in the lobby and said, "We cannot support Priymak's lab. The place is an unmitigated disaster." We were sure that the response would be a strong protest and major objections. Instead, he just said, "OK, no problem." That's one of Goldfarb's charms: He is smart. He instantly recognized that Priymak should not be supported, and he immediately went on to the next step, even though it was obvious that he and Soros were going to have to backtrack from their very public previous announcement.

Goldfarb drove us to the restaurant, where we met the rest of the party. We had an elegant dinner—Goldfarb, Ponomarenko, Priymak, his deputy, the translator, Hale, Salfinger, and me. The food was continental and delicious. The conversation was a triumph of small talk, all through the interpreter. At last, the dreaded moment came. Priymak asked what we thought of his program. We said that it had some good points and some points that could be strengthened. We never gave him a straight answer as to whether the Priymak institute had been approved or disapproved.

Goldfarb later told Priymak that the program had been restructured and that he wasn't going to get the $1.5 million. At the suggestion of Vladimir Starodubov, the deputy health minister, Goldfarb offered Priymak a consolation prize of $150,000 for new equipment, but made it contingent on Priymak's publicly accepting the international comprehensive standard TB therapy, DOTS. He told Priymak, "We can't fund your institute, because it is not in agreement with world TB policies. We would be ostracized." Priymak told him he'd think about it, but never responded.

About 2 years later, Priymak's successor, Professor Mikhail Perelman, approached Goldfarb and asked why he was providing Soros funds to Khomenko's institute and not to the Priymak institute. Goldfarb explained that Khomenko was acceptable to the global TB community, worked with the World Health Organization, and publicly advocated the DOTS strategy. Goldfarb said, "If you as the new director of the Priymak institute join the DOTS club and abandon your harmful policies, I'll be glad to work with you. I can't work with your institute when it's perceived as a bastion of harmful policies." Goldfarb said that Perelman went away promising to think about it, but nothing more was heard.

Our decision to recommend not funding Priymak left a lot of money unspent. Goldfarb ultimately convinced Soros that the funds could be used to control tuberculosis in the prisons, where it was becoming an epidemic. This was the beginning of the Soros-funded effort by the Public Health Research Institute to reverse the disaster of Russian TB control in prisons, for which. Soros later raised his donation to $12 million.

Hot September

The regular summit meeting of the U.S. and Russian vice presidents was coming up. Al Gore of the United States and Viktor Chernomyrdin of Russia and their staffs met regularly to discuss issues of mutual concern. Like most meetings of important politicians, this one was well planned, and there were to be no surprises.

Before the meeting of the Gore-Chernomyrdin commission, Goldfarb got in touch with an old friend he had known since high school, Masha Lipman, who was deputy editor of *Itogi*, a weekly Russian news magazine that was then linked to *Newsweek*. He told her that there was a powerful story about the disastrous and increasing TB epidemic in Russia. He suggested that the story might be tied to the coming Gore-Chernomyrdin meeting, which would include a discussion of health issues. Lipman had just the right reporter for the story—a young woman named Masha Gessen. When she was a teenager, Gessen and her family had moved from Russia to the United States, where she had graduated from an American university. Feeling ties to her homeland, she moved back to Russia as a young adult. Gessen was brilliant, fluent in both English and Russian, and very interested in health stories. She had covered the New York City tuberculosis epidemic in the early 1990s, and she was aware of the disastrous link between AIDS and tuberculosis.

Masha Gessen was delighted to do the story, and she did a terrific job. It was the cover story when *Itogi* hit the newsstands in early September 1997. The headline said: "Tuberculosis: The Triumphant March of Once-Defeated Scourge." Gessen's powerful story described the World Health Organization's strategy of diagnosis and treatment and explained that the Russian method "is diametrically opposed to nearly all of the recommendations embodied in the WHO's approach." Furthermore, Gessen reported that on government orders, doctors in the former Soviet Union had been lying for years about the number of cases of TB. They had reported a steady decline in TB cases, giving figures that were 25 or 30 percent lower than the real numbers. Until recently, they had ignored the number of cases in the prison system, where the TB epidemic was at its worst.

Almost everybody attending the Gore-Chernomyrdin commission had read the story or heard about it. In that heated September atmosphere in Moscow, a city with little or no air-conditioning, the U.S. delegation consisted of Gore, Dr. Donna Shalala, Secretary of the U.S. Department of Health and Human Services, and other health experts, including Abbey Gardner from the Open Society Institute, or Soros Foundation.

Shalala knew that the U.S. government was concerned about the TB epidemic in Russia and that some people were beginning to consider it a threat to U.S. national security. The problem had been raised in previous Gore-Chernomrydin commission meetings. Shalala was also aware that the Russian "TB lobby" opposed Western methods of diagnosis and treatment. But this time Shalala surprised the Soros Foundation team by asking members to give the U.S. delegation a breakfast briefing about the Russian tuberculosis problem the day before the U.S. group met the Russians in formal sessions. In that briefing, Gardner explained that the PHRI/Soros group's work in Russia was built on the DOTS strategy, which the World Health Organization and the major international TB agencies had endorsed as the best way to control and cure tuberculosis. She explained that the Russian Ministry of Health had always resisted DOTS. Gardner pointed out that the ministry was struggling to maintain a huge, outdated national TB infrastructure that included X-rays of the entire population every other year, more than 100 TB sanatoriums, and thousands of TB doctors, thoracic surgeons, nurses, and other personnel.

Shalala listened carefully but didn't indicate what, if anything, she would do. The next day, at the formal meeting of the Health Commission, which she cochaired with her opposite number, Russian Minister of Health Tatyana Dmitriyeva, she asked for a description of the Soros anti-TB program. Then she pointedly asked why Russia was not promoting DOTS as the World Health Organization recommended and as the PHRI/Soros anti-TB program was. Priymak, who was present as Russia's chief TB doctor and the representative to the Gore-Chernomyrdin commission on TB, was the first to respond. He blew up, growing emotional as he explained his opposition to the program of the Soros group, the Public Health Research Institute, and the whole idea of DOTS and its core element, directly observed therapy. He said that Russia had always had the best TB program in the world and that directly observed therapy wasn't needed. He said that the Soros people did not know what they were talking about and that they were roaming around Russia and doing things without consulting with the Ministry of Health. He called it an insult to Russia. It was the only heated discussion of the day.

Shalala was diplomatic, but she said that she supported the Soros Foundation's approach of showing a successful therapy that could be an addition to the existing system, without any insult to anyone. Immediately, Deputy Minister of Health Vladimir Starodubov and Minister Dmitriyeva rejected any criticism of the Soros group, welcomed its work in Russia, and said they completely agreed with the project and supported it.

Priymak left the meeting at the coffee break and didn't come back.

As the months wore on, the Russians feared that Priymak's opposition might antagonize George Soros. They had hoped that Soros would invest hundreds of millions of dollars in the economy, and they didn't want to offend him over a minor matter like arguments over the best treatment for tuberculosis. In early February 1998, the first deputy prime minister, Anatoly Chubais, ordered Priymak's dismissal.

Before he departed, Priymak left his own timebomb behind. He was instrumental in the publication on February 2, 1998, of Prikaz 33 (Order 33) of the Ministry of Health of the Russian Federation.[1] This order, signed by Minister of Health Dmitriyeva, set forth official guidelines on the treatment of tuberculosis. It was binding on all Russian health administrators and was to be used as the framework for managing TB patients and for licensing medical activity against TB. In other words, it was the *law* for treating TB in Russia. What a law it was! All patients with tuberculosis bacteria in their sputum had to be hospitalized for at least 8 weeks. In addition to giving standard anti-TB drugs as pills, doctors could spray drugs directly into TB cavities in the lung or introduce the drugs by puncturing the patient's chest or threading a catheter into the cavity. The standard course of this extraordinary and painful treatment was 10 administrations over 3 or 4 weeks; the course could be repeated. Doctors could also add "pathogenetic therapy," a kind of supportive treatment. It included the use of steroids and vitamin E in an attempt to speed healing and reduce scarring. Surgery could also be used, especially for tuberculosis outside the lungs. There was also a category of TB patients called "chronics," who had frequent relapses.

This extraordinary shopping list leaves Western TB experts shaking their heads in amazement. Seldom is it necessary to hospitalize TB patients, unless they are desperately ill with long-neglected TB. If they have spread the disease to family members or coworkers, they've done it before they got sick enough to be hospitalized. There is no reason to spray or inject TB drugs into the lungs. All these drugs are extremely well absorbed when given as pills. Spraying or injecting them doesn't add anything except the risk of infection and irritation. Giving steroids may slightly speed up the healing of a lung lesion, but the outcome is the same at the end of treatment. Steroids have serious side effects—they reduce the body's ability to fight off many infections, including tuberculosis, and they weaken the bones. There's no evidence that giving vitamins helps TB patients, although it—like TLC (tender loving care)—can't hurt. Western physicians hardly ever need to resort to surgery to treat TB; it is a last, desperate measure in patients whose TB is not curable with any combination of the many drugs in our medicine chest. As for "chronic" TB patients, the Western experts rec-

ognized that many of them probably had multi-drug-resistant TB as a result
of inadequate or inappropriate treatment, or lack of adherence. Good TB
treatment programs do not produce "chronics." And such a category of
patient hardly exists outside Russia. Thanks to Priymak, the Russian archaic
legacy of TB treatment was now written in stone for all Russian physicians.
Doctors who wanted to use faster, cheaper outpatient treatment that had
been shown in the West to be easier on patients would have to get a special exemption from Prikaz 33.

The Secret White House Meeting

Goldfarb was becoming more and more concerned about the tuberculosis problem that was brewing in the Russian prisons. As the Russian economy deteriorated after the breakup of the Soviet Union in 1991, petty
crime escalated. There was no bail; people who had been arrested for minor
crimes were held in pretrial detention centers for months or years, often
without medical attention and in extremely crowded conditions where
transmission of any disease—let alone an airborne disease like tuberculosis—was almost guaranteed. If prisoners with TB got any treatment at all,
it was likely to be poor or chaotic treatment that usually converted ordinary, treatable TB into deadly multi-drug-resistant TB. Prisoners got the
wrong drugs, or they got the right drugs but not enough of them for long
enough, or their treatment program got lost in the shuffle as they were
transferred from one place to another. The Russian prison system held less
than 1 percent of the population (although that was a tremendously high
percentage), but it held close to half the country's TB patients. Goldfarb
put together an appeal to President Boris Yeltsin from the Public Health
Research Institute of New York and two other international nongovernmental aid organizations, Médecins sans Frontières (Doctors without
Borders), a Belgian group, and Medical Emergency Relief International
(MERLIN), a British group. It said:

"Dear Mr. President, We are writing to bring to your attention the alarming situation with the incidence of multi-drug-resistant tuberculosis (MDR-
TB) in the Russian Federation, particularly in its penal system. Our three
non-governmental organizations have been carrying out humanitarian programs aimed to control TB in several regions of Russia. Based on this experience we feel that the issue of MDR-TB is not given appropriate attention
by official health care agencies and prison administration. This neglect, in
our view, may lead to the epidemic getting out of control and indeed becoming unmanageable. . . . "

The letter went on to explain that MDR-TB was caused by misuse of antibiotics in the Russian health-care system, particularly in prisons. Tens of thousands of Russians were getting substandard treatment, the letter said. The criminal justice system needed a reliable supply of antituberculosis drugs, prohibition of substandard TB treatment, and funding for better diagnostic methods and training of personnel.

"Unless these measures are urgently taken," the letter continued, "the epidemic of MDR-TB will spread beyond the confines of the Russian penal system and will cause countless loss of life and enormous economic damage in the Russian society and the world at large in the coming decade."

The letter to Yeltsin got front-page attention in the Russian press, but not even a yawn from Yeltsin. Some establishment organizations felt that Goldfarb had gone too far and been too confrontational—just the sort of behavior you would expect from a former dissident. Nevertheless, it was clear that tuberculosis spreading from Russia was a potential threat to world stability and to national security in the United States. It could appropriately be compared to germ warfare.

Goldfarb mentioned his concerns to Soros, and Soros talked to First Lady Hillary Clinton in the summer of 1998, when the Clintons were vacationing in Southampton, the exclusive resort 100 miles east of New York City on Long Island. Soros told Clinton about the exploding TB problem in Russia and how it posed a threat to everyone.

Very discreetly, on October 28, 1998, Hillary Clinton convened an unprecedented White House meeting on the threat of tuberculosis. There was no publicity, in dramatic contrast to that morning, when the media had swarmed over the White House to cover President Bill Clinton's meeting on AIDS.

Hillary Clinton's meeting included many of the movers and shakers who might have some potential concern or involvement with global aspects of the spread of TB. In addition to Soros and Shalala, those present were Dr. Gro Harlem Bruntland, a physician who had served as prime minister of Norway and now was director general of the World Health Organization; Tom Loftus, the World Health Organization representative in Washington; James Wolfensohn, president of the World Bank; U.S. Agency for International Development (USAID) administrator Brian Atwood; Dr. Margaret Hamburg, assistant secretary for planning and evaluation at the Department of Health and Human Services, who had led New York City's triumph over a TB epidemic in the early 1990s; Dr. Srdjan Matic, medical director of Soros's Open Society Institute; Dr. Paul Farmer, a Harvard professor and activist for human rights who was working to control multi-drug-resistant TB in Peru and Haiti;

Leo Fuerth, national security adviser to Al Gore; and Ken Bernard, from the National Security Council.

In the early afternoon, this impressive group gathered in the Blue Room in the East Wing of the White House. The principals sat around a huge square table, three to a side. Another 20 or so people, including Goldfarb, sat on chairs around this ornate room with its gilded wooden chandelier, marble fireplace, and three long windows offering views of the Washington Monument and the Jefferson Memorial.

Hillary Clinton spoke first. She had been very well briefed and talked in a relaxed manner. Tuberculosis was an international problem, she said, and here were the main players. She turned the floor over to Shalala. According to *TB Monitor*, which reported on the proceedings, Shalala said that the TB threat was global and that if TB was to be controlled in the United States, more attention needed to be paid to controlling it internationally, particularly in Russia. Atwood of USAID agreed that TB in Russia needed attention and that Russia should be urged to comply with the World Health Organization's DOTS strategy. Bruntland said that even though DOTS was the global standard of treatment, it failed to address the problem of multi-drug-resistant TB and was a labor-intensive method that required careful surveillance. She described the World Health Organization's broad Stop TB Initiative. Wolfensohn said that the World Bank had given $300 million to 20 countries in the previous 10 years to help control TB. He praised Soros's efforts against TB in Russia.

Everyone had been well prepared by their staffs. There are seldom surprises at meetings like this. People spoke of their concerns, of the need for the World Bank to follow the lead of the World Health Organization. It was all in abstract, international terms. Russia was, thus far, only a minor part of the discussion.

Then Soros spoke up. He had been getting bored. "I really want to talk about TB in Russia," he said. He said that the TB epidemic there was much worse than people had originally thought. He wanted the World Health Organization to put treatment of multi-drug-resistant tuberculosis on its agenda, a topic many experts thought the organization had been trying to ignore. He asked the World Health Organization to convene a donors' conference, where nations and organizations would commit to funding for TB treatment and eradication in Russia. Hillary Clinton pointed out that Bruntland was seated in the right place, between the financier George Soros and the World Bank president James Wolfensohn. But it seemed to several observers that Bruntland was more interested in the World Health Organization's global Stop TB Initiative, which did not concentrate on Russia.

The results of the meeting were helpful but not spectacular. The World Bank sent a mission to Russia, the first exploration of a possible loan to combat TB in that country. The U.S. Agency for International Development (USAID) contributed a bit more money for its project in Russia. Hillary Clinton's meeting had been a well-planned first step. Though it did not lead to immediate, worldwide action against the world's most common killer infectious disease, it did raise awareness of the global threat of tuberculosis and it certainly brought the right people together. And, it may have been the first time the word *tuberculosis* was mentioned in the White House.

End-of-the-Millennium Report

By 1998 it was clear that multi-drug-resistant tuberculosis was a growing problem around the world. The World Health Organization and the International Union against Tuberculosis and Lung Disease had released a study the year before that identified "hot spots" with high levels of multi-drug-resistant TB: countries of the former Soviet Union, Argentina, one province in China, the Ivory Coast, the Dominican Republic, and one state in India.[2]

Soros's Open Society Institute commissioned Harvard Medical School's Department of Social Medicine to study the problem. Two Harvard physicians, Paul Farmer and Jim Kim, with the help of many others who were active in the global TB arena, put together a massive report, titled *The Global Impact of Drug-Resistant Tuberculosis*,[3] which spelled out in horrific detail the problem in Russia; in many of the other countries of the former Soviet Union; in South Africa, where it was disastrously tied in with the HIV epidemic; and in Peru, where Farmer and Kim had led a successful and continuing effort to treat multi-drug-resistant tuberculosis in the slums of Lima.

Exactly 1 year after the White House meeting, sitting between Soros and the head of the Russian prison system, General Vladimir Yalunin, at the press conference introducing the *Global Impact* report on October 28, 1999, Aryeh Neier, the president of the Open Society Institute, said, "This epidemic will only briefly remain local. It will not remain within borders."

Multi-drug-resistant TB spreads the same way regular TB does—through the air. It travels with people, whether they are government officials, investment bankers, smugglers, or illegal immigrants. After the collapse of the Soviet Union, when restrictions were relaxed, travel between Russia and the rest of the world skyrocketed. About 3 million tourists traveled from Russia to Europe alone in 1998. Millions more crossed the borders for reasons other than tourism.

Already, the *Global Impact* report said, all the nations bordering Russia had reported cases of TB in immigrants or travelers from Russia. In the countries along the Baltic, multi-drug-resistant strains of tuberculosis similar to those in Russia had been identified. The same multi-drug-resistant strains had shown up among immigrants from the former Soviet Union to Germany, Israel, and the United States. Drug-resistant cases had increased by 50 percent in Denmark and Germany.[4] A conference of British health experts had concluded that London could experience a tuberculosis epidemic similar to the one that New York had in the late 1980s and early 1990s.[5]

Farmer, the lead author of the report, stressed that the World Health Organization's DOTS strategy must be used, together with a program offering second-line drugs for people with multi-drug-resistant TB. He explained that DOTS works only for people with drug-sensitive TB; when TB is already drug-resistant, DOTS can actually promote more drug resistance. In Lima, Peru, he and his colleague Dr. Jim Kim had seen that DOTS was failing in a community where multi-drug-resistant TB was common. They began testing patients for drug resistance and treating them with the expensive second-line drugs to which their TB was sensitive. With perseverance and by cajoling drug manufacturers and distributors, Farmer and Kim managed to get the second-line drugs somewhat more cheaply. They were beginning to succeed in saving lives and stopping the spread of multi-drug-resistant TB.

There was a new name for their program, coined by Dr. Arata Kochi, then head of the World Health Organization's Stop TB Initiative. He was the first to call Farmer and Kim's program "DOTS-Plus." The new name has stuck.

The *Global Impact* report got a lot of attention. The *New York Times* carried a long story by Judith Miller, "Study Says New TB Strains Need an Intensive Strategy."[6] The *Boston Globe*, the Associated Press, Reuters, and a German news agency also carried major stories.

The proposed "intensive strategy" to treat patients with multi-drug-resistant TB was going to cost money, estimated at that time as perhaps as much as $1 billion. Multi-drug-resistant tuberculosis demands attention, said Aryeh Neier. "TB is not like Ebola or AIDS, that spread through close contact. TB spreads through the air." As Richard Bumgarner said some years ago, "Tuberculosis is Ebola with wings!"

6

Inside the Gulag

In September 1998, just a year after our eye-opening evaluation of the Priymak institute in Moscow, I made another trip to Russia. This time I saw just what Russian prisons were like, and why they were culturing, promoting, and spreading tuberculosis and its more deadly multi-drug-resistant form. This time I traveled to deepest Siberia to visit prisons and prison TB colonies as chairman of the advisory committee on Russian TB programs of the Public Health Research Institute (PHRI). Our committee's job was to assess several anti-TB programs funded by George Soros's $12 million grant to Alex Goldfarb and his PHRI's TB project in Russia. This grant was an increase from his aborted $1.5 million donation to fund the Priymak institute's TB laboratory. Our committee would also make recommendations to the Moscow office of the U.S. Agency for International Development about using its funds for TB projects. We were going to look at programs in prisons and the civilian sector in two areas of the Kemerovo region in western Siberia, which has three pretrial detention centers, 28 prison colonies with 30,000 inmates, and two special TB colonies for prisoners with active TB.

Along with Goldfarb and me were a distinguished group of experts: Dr. Rick O'Brien, the director of research and evaluation of the Tuberculosis Elimination Division of the U.S. Centers for Disease Control and Prevention; Dr. Barry Kreiswirth, a well-known microbiologist at the Public Health Research Institute, who had identified the multi-drug-resistant strain that was responsible for much of the MDR-TB emergency in New York in the early 1990s; Dr. Malgosia Grzemska, the World Health Organization's representative for tuberculosis programs in eastern Europe, Russia, and the former Soviet Union; Dr. Naomi Bock, an infectious disease physician, and expert on TB in prisons, who was then on the faculty at Emory University in Atlanta; Dr. Michael Kimerling of the University of Alabama, an international expert in prison health and TB; Dr. Alex Sloutsky, a microbiologist from the Massachusetts Department of Health; Dr. Paul Farmer, a physician-anthropologist from Partners in Health, a nongovernmental organization affiliated with the Department of Social Medicine at Harvard Medical School; and Dr. Max Salfinger, the New York State mycobacteriology laboratory director, who had accompanied me on the visit to the Priymak institute the year before.

I've spent my career working with TB patients, who are often on the margins of society, but nothing had prepared me for what I saw in Siberia. The Russian criminal justice system is vastly different from any in the West. After someone is arrested for a crime, he (it's usually a man) is held first in a holding cell in a police station, and then in a pretrial detention center called a SIZO (from its initials in Russian). He can be held in the SIZO for as long as 5 years, although the average seems to be about a year. During that time, the detainees are shuttled back and forth from the SIZO to court, often over long distances (sometimes hundreds or thousands of miles) for days or weeks. After trial and conviction—and most people are convicted—they are sent to prisons (which are labor colonies), usually for a term of 4 years.[1] Conditions in SIZOs as well as in prisons are frightening, as we were discovering, and they are ideal not only for spreading TB but also for fostering drug-resistant strains. Malnutrition is common among inmates, which is not surprising given that the prison system spends only about $26 a year on caring for each prisoner.[2] In most SIZOs, healthy inmates are seldom separated from those with TB.

The Kemerovo prison was the worst I had ever seen. In a typical cell, 30 prisoners were crowded into one room, and the only toilet was a hole in the corner. Since there were only 10 beds, the 30 prisoners had to sleep in shifts. The ones who weren't sleeping lounged about the cell or sat on the floor. Many of them were coughing, and, since this was Siberia and winter was coming on, there was no fresh air. The windows were sealed, as they would be until spring. Heavy shutters shut out sunlight and air. The prisoners had no uniforms but wore their own tattered clothing. Their laundry was strung on clotheslines, and the damp clothing contributed to the heavy air, which was invariably hazy with cigarette smoke as well. The prisoners' meager belongings hung in plastic shopping bags at the ends of the triple-tiered beds that they shared in shifts. For meals, an attendant came around with a bucket of soup, which he ladled into the prisoners' own well-worn bowls. The soup, plus a piece of tough black bread, was all they got to eat —no milk or eggs or meat, no fruit or vegetables, just soup and black bread. I couldn't tell what the soup was. I suspect they couldn't either.

I will never forget the clang of the heavy iron door that let my team out to freedom and kept those prisoners in. The sound reverberates in my head to this day.

Overcrowding in SIZOs and prisons reaches extraordinary levels. Crammed into a room of about 80 square meters (or about 860 square feet) will be perhaps 80 prisoners, 30 or 40 bunk beds stacked along the side walls, and a long table and two benches down the center.[3] This is about 10 square feet per prisoner. In the United States, a single prisoner is allotted 80 square feet.[4] To think of Russian prison space in familiar terms, consider that the prison unit is about 20 by 40 feet, the size of a living room plus a family room or dining room, or of an office conference room. It holds 80 human beings, closed in day and night, winter and summer.

Whenever I entered a cell in Siberia, I wore a duckbill mask (an N95 respirator certified by the U.S. National Institute of Occupational Safety and Health). I had never used any mask before in my life, but on this trip, because of the astounding prevalence of multi-drug-resistant TB, I insisted that everybody on my team wear one. I had brought the masks in my hand luggage to make sure they wouldn't get lost.

Masks are a great nuisance, but the U.S. Occupational Safety and Health Administration (OSHA) requires all U.S. health personnel working with TB patients to wear them, after onerous and expensive "fit testing" to ensure a tight seal around the nose and mouth. The N95 respirators look like ordinary surgical masks, except that the area over the mouth extends in a flat, orange-colored fold like a duck's bill. Though they probably create an effective barrier to organisms such as TB bacteria, they're so silly looking that they also create an unfortunate barrier to communication between the doctor and the vulnerable, frightened patient.

My opinion, not very popular with OSHA, is that using such a mask simply doesn't make sense most of the time. Tuberculosis is almost invariably spread by the patient who hasn't yet been diagnosed. Once it's known that a patient has TB, he or she will be given medication and probably will very quickly become noninfectious. But in the United States, OSHA rules require medical professionals to wear masks with all *already diagnosed* TB patients, under penalty of major financial sanctions to their medical centers. It would make more sense to insist that all people in the emergency room or even the diabetic clinic—receptionists, clerks, nurses, doctors, technicians, and housekeepers—wear masks. In the emergency room, people are coughing and no one knows what they've got. A cardinal rule of TB care has always been that "the dangerous case is the *undiagnosed* case."

Do the Numbers

Tuberculosis is so common in Russia's enormous prison system that Alex Goldfarb believes, probably correctly, that almost everyone who has spent time in a Russian detention center or prison has either latent or active tuberculosis.[5] The prison system holds about 1 million prisoners. About 10 percent of them have active, usually infectious, tuberculosis, and most of the rest have latent TB infection without active TB, but they have a 10 percent lifetime risk of progressing to active TB. Obviously the likelihood of infection increases with each day a healthy prisoner is incarcerated in close quarters with infectious prisoners. About one-third of the prisoners with active TB have multi-drug-resistant TB. The death rate among prisoners is 30 times higher than that among TB patients in the general population.[6]

Of the 300,000 people released from the Russian prison system each year, the best guess is that 30,000 of them have *active* TB (not a latent infection), and at least 10,000 of those 30,000 probably have multi-drug-resistant TB. Because of overcrowding, amnesties are frequent. The most recent, in late 2000, sent an additional 140,000 prisoners, many of them probably with active TB, out into the communities across Russia. Each year, about 300,000 new prisoners come into the prison system, where they will experience the same dreadful conditions and will probably be infected with TB and multi-drug-resistant TB.

It is no wonder that TB experts call the Russian prison system a pump that spews TB into Russia's towns and cities, and then to countries that were formerly part of the Soviet Union, like Latvia and Estonia, to Western countries like Finland and Denmark, and around the world through the magic of fast airline transportation.

The Russian Legal System

Russia won admission to the Council of Europe in 1997 on condition that it reform its criminal justice system. In 1998, the administration of Russia's prisons was transferred from the Ministry of the Interior to the Ministry of Justice.[7] While the Ministry of Justice is making efforts to reform the system, it faces a severe uphill battle. In Soviet times, the prisons were the Gulag, which is the name still used by most people: a chain of prison labor camps. Today they are part of GUIN, the State Administration for the Carrying Out of Punishment, a division of the Ministry of Justice.

Almost 1 percent of the population of Russia is imprisoned, a higher percentage than in any other nation in the world. (The United States comes second.) There are several reasons for this, as we learned on our visit. After the economic collapse in 1991, there was an increase in petty crime, such as burglaries, stealing cars, snatching handbags, and pickpocketing. Russia has a harsh penal code, a legacy of czarist and Stalinist times, with long sentences for relatively minor crimes. For example, a 14-year-old boy got 6 years for stealing a crate of vodka with two buddies.[8] A student who got drunk and assaulted a man "got 8 years for two punches and two rubles," according to Andrei Babushkin, head of a civil rights organization.[9]

Until very recently there was no bail in Russia. Even now, less than 2 percent of people arrested are released on bail while they await trial; and most of those are mobsters with easy access to bribe money.[10] Dr. Andrew Coyle, director of the International Centre for Prison Studies at King's College, London, and former head of Brixton Prison in London, says that the chief prosecutor of one of the countries of the former Soviet Union was astounded to hear that many people who were put on trial in the United Kingdom were found innocent and released; in his system fewer than 1 percent were ever found innocent. The Soviet prosecutor, according to Coyle, "was aghast: 'But that means you are detaining innocent people!'" The assumption was that only guilty people were arrested in the Soviet Union.[11]

Occasionally, if there are facilities for it in the SIZO, inmates may be X-rayed for TB and tested for HIV.[12] Prisoners who are diagnosed with active tuberculosis may be isolated in a cell with other prisoners with TB and treated with isoniazid and rifampin, assuming that the drugs are available. Since no drug susceptibility studies are done, this is a perfect way to create multi-drug-resistant tuberculosis. (Multi-drug-resistant tuberculosis is defined as TB resistant to isoniazid and rifampin, the most powerful and effective drugs used to treat TB.) When a prisoner whose TB bacteria have unsuspected resistance to rifampin is treated with rifampin and isoniazid, the bacteria will quickly learn how to become resistant to isoniazid. If his bacteria are resistant to isoniazid, they will learn how to become resistant to rifampin. And then he'll pass those multi-drug-resistant bacteria on—to whomever he shares the air with.

The SIZOs

My team wasn't alone in recognizing the dreadful conditions in Russia's SIZOs and prisons. They have been described by several Western journalists and prison experts. Even a Russian government official lamented the problem. "You can't help but feel for a girl of 18 who is waiting in a pretrial detention center for the third year because she stole a fur coat," Justice

Minister Pavel Krasheninnikov told Reuters, saying that he was deeply concerned about the conditions in Russian pretrial detention centers and prisons. He said he hoped to limit pretrial detention to 1 year for adults and 6 months for youths.[13]

The *New York Times* reported that "inside Matrosskya Tishina [a major detention center in Moscow], where 5000 prisoners are held in a prison built for 2000, lies a Dickensian world of filth, squalor and disease. Inside fetid, windowless cells, prisoners are covered in lice. Rats dart out of the walls. Prisoners stretch out tin bowls through a tiny opening in the door to receive bread and a gloopy gruel of kasha, or buckwheat, that is served for breakfast, lunch and dinner. The exercise yards are cement rooms in the attic, where prisoners can see the sky by squinting through a webbed roof of barbed wire."[14]

The pretrial detention centers are far more crowded than the prisons. A U.N. special representative on torture, Sir Nigel Rodley, also visited Matrosskaya Tishina and reported,

"Due to overcrowding . . . there is insufficient room for everyone to lie down, sit down or even stand up at the same time. . . . All the detainees in these cells suffer from swollen feet and legs due to the fact that they must stand for extensive periods of time. The inmates tend to be half-clothed and are even stripped to their undershirts (at least in summer . . .). Their bodies are perspiring and nothing can dry due to the humidity. . . . The cells are disease incubators."[15]

Disease incubators indeed, when the disease is like tuberculosis, which spreads through the air. The infectious droplets can hang for a long time in damp, dark conditions. Sunlight ordinarily kills the bacteria, and breezes of fresh air will sweep them outside, where they will be dispersed and killed. But in these prisons and SIZOs there is no light and no fresh air, so the TB bacteria persist in the air, waiting to be breathed in.

In Russia, TB experts report, "In many pre-trial detention centers, every cell contains at least one prisoner with active pulmonary TB. TB infection control measures . . . have been rendered irrelevant in the context of massive overcrowding. Even if adequate ventilation and [artificial] ultraviolet lights [which have the same TB-killing effect as sunlight] were installed universally, it is likely that such measures would be rendered ineffective in the face of such high levels of exposure."

Many prison health officials and international observers have concluded that a large majority of detainees—more than 80 percent, in the opinion of the Public Health Research Institute—are infected with latent but viable

M. tuberculosis.[16] In comparison, fewer than 10 percent of U.S. prisoners have latent TB infection.

Medical care is usually not available in the holding cells in the police stations. Some care is provided in SIZOs, but it is usually erratic, and a reliable supply of any needed drugs is lacking. Although conditions could not be better for spreading tuberculosis, people held in SIZOs cannot be transferred to the special "TB colonies" until they are sentenced.[17] Since most people who are arrested are convicted (months to years later), most are then sent to a prison colony, often far away. Patients with TB are not segregated from healthy prisoners on the journey there.

The Russian Attitude to Imprisonment

In the West, people think that, ideally, prison should help to reform the convict. Training courses, learning a trade, and counseling are ways to help the prisoner become a law-abiding person who may some day be able to rejoin the community, notes Coyle.[18] But Russians have a different view. In the days of the czars and Stalin, dissidents, criminals, and difficult intellectuals were exiled to Siberia. After completing their sentences, many exiles stayed in communities near the prison. In czarist times they were often forbidden to go back home. Today, released prisoners may not have the money to pay for a trip home.

Coyle writes, "Imprisonment in the countries of the Soviet Union was based on a different set of principles [from those in the West]. Prisoners were enemies of the state. They were literally outlaws, placed outside the law. One thing which the state could demand from them in return was labour. This was added on to the Tsarist notion of exile to far-flung parts of the Empire. The sentence was still to be served in Siberia but now it also included a requirement to work for the state."[19]

In Soviet times, Coyle explains, the prisons were self-supporting industrial factories, and prisoners worked long shifts. In this complex system, prison factories in one region produced parts for prison factories in another region, and vice versa. After the Soviet Union disintegrated into separate nations, however, this industrial prison system collapsed, and living conditions for the prisoners went from bad to worse. Today the prisons generate little if any income. Instead of being self-supporting, they need money from Russia or from one of the newly independent countries to pay guards, to pay for food, to buy supplies, to keep the heat and lights on, and to buy medicines for sick inmates. But, in these post-Soviet hard times, money is difficult to find, and even when it is available, prisons are not a priority. Thus the prisons often run low on food and more often run out of medicines. Furthermore, the prisoners have nothing to do any more. They remain in their overcrowded, airless cells, instead of marching out to the factory every day.

TB Colony 33

The best care for prisoners with TB, inadequate as it often is, is provided in the system's special TB colonies. If a prisoner is diagnosed with TB, he is supposed to be sent to a special TB colony. However, since these are usually at double or triple capacity, sick prisoners often remain in the regular prison with healthy inmates. We found this to be the case when we got to TB Colony 33 in Mariinsk, which is either a hell hole or the first sign of hope, depending on how you look at it.

Mariinsk is a small town in the Kemerovo region. It's a 4-hour drive from Kemerovo city along a two-lane road that is steeply canted so that the heavy snows of winter can be plowed off to the side. Although the Kemerovo region is a center of coal mining, the road to Mariinsk goes through pleasant farms and forests of tall, thin, silver birch trees.

TB Colony 33 is where prisoners with TB are transferred from other prisons in the region. It has 750 beds and more than 1300 patients.[20] TB Colony 33's heroine is its chief physician, Dr. Natalya Vezhnina, a small dynamo with short blonde hair and a lively smile. She wears a neat olive-green uniform with gold stars on the shoulders and a shirt and tie, because she is a colonel in GUIN, the prison administration.

"In 1990," she told the *Moscow Times*, "I had medicine and things were all right. I had nearly 2000 patients and 16 to 20 died each year. I knew all their names. By 1992 it became very difficult. Already 60 people died that year. I had no medicine, not even aspirin to treat a headache. Then it became worse and I never knew any of their names. It is terrible to see people die and not be able to do anything."[21] By then, hundreds were dying.

With the approval of her boss, Vezhnina went to a human rights convention in Moscow. She appealed for foreign help. According to *Newsweek*, she said, "I have a real prison where real people are dying of a real disease. If any of you can help, I'll welcome you with open arms."

Médecins sans Frontières (Doctors without Borders) came to help in 1995, bringing in a young team of doctors, nurses, and lab technicians from Belgium. When they arrived, they found corpses stacked in the corridors and in the showers, awaiting autopsies, which would inevitably show that they had died of TB. Three or four people were dying each day.[22] The team was headed by Dr. Hans Kluge; Dr. Michael Kimerling served as a consultant. Médecins sans Frontières used many foreign experts, although they also worked with the local staff. While this method may work well when the foreign team is present, some feel there is a risk that things will deteriorate when the foreigners ultimately leave. Unfortunately, most programs supported by donor organizations are likely to suffer the same problem. Nevertheless, this was considered by most to be a top-notch operation. The Belgian team used the Department of Microbiology at the highly respected Institute of Tropical Medicine in Antwerp, a World Health Organization reference laboratory, to check their lab results. It was a very promising start.

With considerable difficulty and many negotiations, they arranged for a supply of reliable drugs manufactured in Europe. Although Russian pharmaceutical firms make TB drugs, they do not yet adhere to the "good manufacturing practices" rules of the U.S. Food and Drug Administration, which include plant inspections, so their quality may not be as trustworthy as it should be; some Russian manufacturers are expected to meet this requirement in the near future. Although a pill may contain the appropriate drug, the drug may not be bioavailable—easily absorbed by the body—and this is a key factor in treatment failure.

The Médecins sans Frontières team knew that the prisoners with TB had been waiting in prisons for months before they were transferred to TB Colony 33 and that most had previously received inadequate treatment with antibiotics. Maybe only one drug had been given, maybe more, or maybe the drugs were given intermittently, depending mainly on what drugs were available instead of on the patient's symptoms[23] and his drug susceptibility profile. The MSF group decided that the best thing to do was to put all the prisoners on the standard five-drug World Health Organization regimen for *previously treated* patients, which included streptomycin. All doses of all drugs were directly observed for the entire 6-month course. The nurses were rigorous: They watched carefully as the prisoners washed down the drugs with a nutritious drink. They checked the prisoners' mouths, hands, and cups to make sure they had indeed swallowed the pills and weren't saving them to sell, hide, or trade within the prison. They took regular sputum samples to look for TB bacteria under the microscope. When the bacteria disappeared, it seemed to them that the patients were on their way to cure, which should be achieved in 6 months. Unfortunately, they did not culture the TB bacteria to test for drug susceptibility, which would have told a different story.

The patients were not on their way to cure. Results were disappointing. In the first group of prisoners, less than half were cured. Here we had a good regimen by Western standards, properly given under directly observed conditions, but more than a third were definite treatment failures. What was going on?

For the next group of patients, the team performed lengthy, complex laboratory tests. They cultured each patient's sputum to grow the TB bacteria. It took several weeks for the sluggish TB bacteria to multiply. Then they did drug-susceptibility testing, another time-consuming process, by culturing each patient's TB bacteria with each of the antibiotics being used. They double-checked their results with the reference laboratory in Antwerp.

The results were astonishing, and far more ominous than anyone had suspected. The Médecins sans Frontières team expected that perhaps 5 percent of their patients at Colony 33 would have multi-drug-resistant TB. They underestimated. Nearly 23 percent of the prisoners had multi-drug-resistant TB *before* they started treatment. Two-thirds of them were resistant to isoniazid. Only one-quarter of the patients were sensitive to all the antibiotics tested.

As hard as this was to fathom, it was evident that adding only one drug (streptomycin) to the standard four-drug regimen for sensitive cases, as recommended by WHO, was making the situation worse. It was increasing drug resistance. When you give a TB patient who is already resistant to several drugs a regimen that includes those drugs and one new one, you encourage the bacteria to become resistant to the newly added drug. Since many of these prisoners already had some drug resistance, despite its best intentions and careful treatment, the Médecins sans Frontières team was actually manufacturing more multi-drug-resistant TB in Colony 33. And when the inmates were released, they were shipping it out to the community: Already 300 patients had been released after completing their sentences. Of equal concern, the staff of Colony 33—the guards, the secretaries, the doctors and nurses—were also continuously exposed to multi-drug-resistant TB, and they went home every night to their families.

Unfortunately, at present there is no coordination between the prisons and civilian TB authorities in most of the Russian villages, towns, and cities to which prisoners are released. Released prisoners are usually told to report to the TB dispensary in their area, but few do. According to Vera Denisova, a Red Cross doctor in the Kemerovo region, many released prisoners stop taking their medications once they are free of the prison's strict control. If their symptoms persist, they may occasionally and sporadically buy one or two medications that are available over the counter from a pharmacy, again, encouraging the development of resistance—and infecting people around them. Denisova estimates that about 9 percent of TB patients (not just prisoners) in Kemerovo have multi-drug-resistant TB and that 17 percent have TB that is resistant to at least one drug.[24]

The Moral Question

Until Dr. Paul Farmer, who was a member of our team visiting prisons in Siberia, came on the TB scene, the World Health Organization and many other public health groups recommended treating TB with cheap, effective DOTS. DOTS is WHO's brand name for the standard, effective, clinically proven four-drug regimen given under specific conditions that is the proposed standard of care around the world. The acronym DOTS, in use since 1995, originally stood for directly observed therapy short-course, but actually, when developed by Karel Styblo of the International Union Against Tuberculosis and Lung Disease, consisted of a menu of five specific elements required for good TB treatment: a national TB control program, laboratory monitoring, directly observed therapy, a reliable and constant drug supply, and good recording and reporting. These elements represent WHO's comprehensive TB control strategy. Unfortunately, the Russian Ministry of Health and many in the Russian health establishment have always officially opposed and derided the WHO DOTS strategy.

If treatment using DOTS didn't work, it meant that the patient likely had multi-drug-resistant TB, and this would be far too expensive and difficult to cure in countries with limited resources. WHO felt that it made far more sense to treat patients with ordinary (drug-sensitive) TB, who could be cured easily. WHO also felt (but didn't state publicly) that the rest would most likely die anyway. Since that was the approved protocol of the World Health Organization and the major international TB organizations, that was the approach adopted by Alex Goldfarb's Public Health Research Institute project and his source of funds, George Soros's Open Society Institute.

Probably none of us then recognized the size of the multi-drug-resistant TB problem or the scary fact that preexisting drug resistance may be amplified by the DOTS regimen. Farmer felt differently. Farmer is a tall, thin, supercharged Harvard physician with a strong interest in human rights. Trained first as an anthropologist and then as a physician, he began working in Haiti, a desperately poor country with no infrastructure to speak of. He founded and still runs a medical center, Zanmi Lasante ("Partners in Health" in Haitian Creole), in Haiti's central plateau, where he manages to treat AIDS patients with the expensive, effective drugs that will prolong their lives. He gets the drugs by begging and negotiating, as was recounted in a profile in *The New Yorker* magazine. Farmer's work has been recognized by a MacArthur Foundation "genius grant," all $220,000 of which he donated to Partners in Health.[25]

Farmer and Dr. Jim Kim, his colleague in Partners in Health, showed the same determination and initiative when they got involved in tuberculosis control and treatment in Peru, which had a lot of TB. About half the cases were concentrated in Carabayllo, a slum on the northern fringe of Peru's capital, Lima. Although the Peruvian national TB program was considered one of the best in the world, it wasn't curing enough patients because many patients had multi-drug-resistant TB even though they had never been treated for TB. That meant that they had caught multi-drug-resistant TB from another person who already had it—a frightening situation. Many doctors would have given up. They would just have followed the WHO protocol and not treated these patients, expecting them to die. Farmer and Kim didn't. They worked with Peruvian TB experts and involved local community people in an exhaustive effort to find and treat people with multi-drug-resistant TB. They arranged for drug-sensitivity testing at the Massachusetts State Laboratory, so that they would know which of the remaining anti-TB drugs would be effective in these patients. They hired people from the community to deliver the drugs to patients and watch them take the pills. Their program of treating multi-drug-resistant TB with individually created regimens on the basis of drug susceptibility laboratory testing—later called DOTS-Plus—saved lives by curing people with multi-drug-resistant TB and thereby preventing its spread.[26]

In Lima, Farmer and Kim were continuing to show that multi-drug-resistant TB could be cured in relatively small numbers of patients. But their experience conflicted with that of the World Health Organization, which had long promoted DOTS but effectively left patients with multi-drug-resistant TB to die. Farmer and Kim argued passionately that people couldn't be left to die of MDR-TB, which they had shown in Peru was a treatable disease, even if curing them was difficult and expensive—an argument we were to hear again in the context of expensive drugs to treat AIDS patients in Africa.

Farmer asked the Open Society Institute for a donation. The institute turned him down on the grounds that it was already supporting Goldfarb's Public Health Research Institute program in Russia, and that that program in Russia was following the WHO recommendation of treating sensitive TB and ignoring MDR-TB.

Farmer wrote Soros an impassioned letter, pleading that the Russian project not abandon people with multi-drug-resistant TB. Soros responded by inviting Famer to a meeting. With Farmer in his office, Soros got Goldfarb on the phone wherever he was—London, Moscow—and yelled at him. Goldfarb yelled back. Soros told Goldfarb that he and Farmer would have to sort out the question of treating multi-drug-resistant TB or there would be *no* money for Goldfarb's Russian anti-TB project. Shortly thereafter, there was a heated meeting of the Public Health Research Institute's advisory committee in New York, with the Paul Farmer-Alex Goldfarb controversy and Soros's financial threat the overriding agenda item. After the meeting, we all adjourned to Keen's Steak House, a dark, woody, nineteenth-century restaurant on West 36th Street. Farmer and Goldfarb continued their acrimonious discussion. Things were not going the way I had hoped. We faced the moral dilemma of treating only ordinary TB versus a more complicated and far more expensive program of treating both ordinary TB and multi-drug-resistant TB. The Soros threat of no more funding was real. I felt that the only way to reconcile the two was to invite Farmer to join the advisory committee on our upcoming September 1998 visit to Siberia, where our team would visit the sites where the Soros/Public Health Research Institute would be working. I figured that a week in Siberia, in relatively close quarters, might help.

That was why Farmer, passionate and argumentative, was with Goldfarb, passionate and argumentative, and the rest of the committee as we visited deplorable prisons full of TB patients in Siberia. Just as in Peru, Farmer expressed his powerful belief that people couldn't be left to die of a treatable disease, even if curing them was difficult and expensive. Treatment for patients with multi-drug-resistant TB had to be offered at the same time as treatment for ordinary TB. Of course, that meant that we'd need sophisticated labs for drug-sensitivity testing. Lima was one thing; there had been perhaps a few hundred patients with multi-drug-resistant TB—Farmer's first and highly successful study involved only 50 patients. Here was Russia, an enormous country stretching across half the globe, with many cities, slums, and prisons where there were untold, unnumbered thousands of patients with multi-drug-resistant TB. Further complicating the issue was Russia's TB establishment, long out of touch with Western advances in treatment, which clung to the old largely unnecessary and ineffective ways.

Farmer and Goldfarb continued arguing during the whole week of the advisory committee's visit to Siberian prisons. Perhaps it was the grim conditions in Siberia, perhaps it was the ample vodka we all shared, but Farmer ultimately won Goldfarb over. Not only that, but this was his first step in turning the whole global TB community around. Less than a year later, Farmer and Kim, with Professor Howard Hiatt, former dean of the Harvard School of Public Health, organized a widely attended meeting at the

American Academy of Arts and Sciences in Cambridge, Massachusetts, to promote treatment of multi-drug-resistant TB and to plan the procurement of second-line drugs. Remarkably, the World Health Organization was reluctantly beginning to agree with Farmer's approach. Dr. Arata Kochi, then the head of the WHO Global Tuberculosis Programme, coined the term *DOTS-Plus* to describe the treatment of patients with multi-drug-resistant TB.

DOTS-Plus required drug-sensitivity testing and tailored treatment with second-line drugs for patients with multi-drug-resistant TB, the method Farmer and Kim had shown to work in Peru. By 1999, WHO had endorsed the concept of DOTS-Plus if it was controlled. Since multi-drug-resistant TB was entirely of human origin, and usually occurred because of poor TB programs, it was clear from the beginning that DOTS-Plus had to be used together with an effective, well-functioning DOTS program for treatment of patients with ordinary drug-sensitive TB. In other words, people had to recognize that a poor treatment program for ordinary TB caused resistance and a good treatment program for ordinary TB had to be established before treatment of drug-resistant TB with DOTS-Plus could be started. By 2000, WHO had organized a protocol requiring official sanctioning that would allow procurement of expensive second-line drugs for effective DOTS-Plus programs around the globe. This "Green Light Committee," hosted by WHO with highly respected assessors from several countries, has proven very effective in moving DOTS-Plus forward.

Hope in Tomsk

One place where TB control seemed to be working well and in a coordinated manner was Tomsk, in Siberia. The Tomsk region is an area the size of Poland with a population of about a million, half of whom live in Tomsk city. In contrast to the popular idea of Siberia as a flat wasteland, Tomsk city is built on hills rising above the wide Tom river. It was an important commercial center and river crossing point in the past; now it has a modern four-lane bridge leading to a major highway and small farms on the other side of the river.

Tomsk is one of the oldest cities in Siberia, founded in 1604. It is home to one of Russia's top universities and medical schools, fostered in the past by dissidents and intellectuals who were "exiled to Siberia." The university is housed in classical buildings on a wooded bluff high above the river. The old part of town is filled with typical Siberian wooden houses with elaborately carved and painted shutters and window trim, a cross between a log cabin and a San Francisco Victorian "painted lady." There are some elegant early-nineteenth-century buildings, a modern theater, touches of art deco on the main street, and spacious squares. The rest of the hilly city is made up of typical Soviet apartment houses, 4 to 20 stories tall, set back from the roads in scraggly, muddy fields decorated with wrecked cars, kiosks selling vodka and snacks, and many, many stray dogs. Huge pipes, perhaps 3 feet in diameter and wrapped in silvery insulation, snake alongside the road, up over railroad tracks, and, downtown, sometimes under the sidewalk. The pipes bring heat from two steam plants to the whole city. They make it possible for some homeless people to live outdoors, sleeping where the pipes go under the sidewalk, even in the frigid Siberian winter. Outside Tomsk city, there are a few small towns, the most prominent being the closed city of Seversk, where nuclear research is carried out. There are also many tiny hamlets reachable only in good weather and often lacking even a feldsher (physician assistant or paramedic) because such positions have been left unfilled for lack of funds.

In 1994, Tomsk had a TB epidemic.[27] In December of that year, the British charity Medical Emergency Relief International (MERLIN) came to help and began to introduce DOTS. By all accounts, the program (which is still in action) worked well. Unfortunately, however, it increased the official Russian rage against DOTS and against "interfering, patronizing" Westerners, because it focused on diagnosis of TB by looking for bacteria under the microscope, not by X-ray, the traditional Russian method. This stubborn attitude, increasingly polarized on both sides, to this day hinders the entire anti-TB program in Russia and complicated lengthy negotiations (they have been going on for 3 years) with the World Bank for a loan to fight TB and with the World Health Organization, which was advising the bank.

In late 1997, the Public Health Research Institute, supported by the enhanced grant from Soros, came to Tomsk to extend MERLIN's successful civilian treatment program to the prisons. Tomsk is the first place in Russia where TB diagnosis, treatment, and follow-up care are coordinated in both the prison and civilian sectors. PHRI tried to make an effort to involve mostly local staff in the work and to train them so that they could take over when the time came for the foreign experts to pull out, but, as in all these programs, one never knows if the a transition to the local experts has been a success or a failure until after the fact.

Regional Coalition to Fight TB

The Tomsk region was fortunate in having a very progressive governor, Viktor M. Kress, who recognized that the old system was not working and was far too expensive. He became a national spokesman for the fight against TB and helped organize the Regional Coalition against TB, an association of 18 governors.

The coalition was announced at a well-attended press conference in Moscow on September 29, 1999. Kress, the regional governors, World Bank officials, and various experts met at the Ministry of Science and Technology of the Russian Federation, a building in the spare 1950s international style. The building, which has a spacious central atriumlike space and a graceful marble staircase leading to pleasant meeting rooms on the second floor, is hidden in a secluded enclave facing a green square tucked behind one of Moscow's main streets. The group gathered around a long table in a high-ceilinged room with wood-paneled walls and large windows looking out on the square. Journalists lined the room, sitting on chairs against the wall.

Dr. Joana Godinho of the World Bank, a slim, dark-haired woman with quiet authority, had the meeting tightly organized. She expressed the hope that this "important initiative" of the regional governors could be expanded to include treatment for HIV and other sexually transmitted diseases and that it would be part of the Russian government's Health Reform Implementation Project, a pilot project begun in 1997. "A TB and AIDS project falls into the larger framework of health reform in Russia," she said. "It is important to focus on this urgent problem in order to prevent these epidemics getting a lot worse. I want to reassure you that you have the support of the World Bank and other donors in the world community."

Governor Kress stressed the importance of setting up the coalition and described the programs in Tomsk, which was already more advanced than the other regions in combating TB. The regional governors spoke of opportunities for combined purchasing of drugs and creation of a patient database so that patients could be followed up and treatment success evaluated, initiatives that would be considered advanced even for some Western TB control programs.

The Russian government had requested a $150 million loan spread over 10 years, $100 million for TB, and $50 million for HIV/AIDS. According to an agreement between the Ministry of Health and the Ministry of Justice, the project would be mounted at the federal level, but the most interest was at the regional level. Regions would be able to compete for funding for various projects. Godinho stressed that in dealing with TB, both the health sector and the prison sector must be integrated. "An important requirement will be political will at the regional level, and local capacity—access to both first- and second-line drugs," she said.

Representatives of several regions told of severe epidemics in their prison systems. One from Sverdlovsk said, "There should be no borders between people, as there are no borders with illness. Out of a population of 4½ million, we have 16,000 citizens with active tuberculosis and over 5000 temporarily isolated from society. I'm talking about those in the penal system. These are nurseries for the dissemination of illness."

Several people at the meeting agreed that the Tomsk experience was important because it demonstrated success with a system that treated both prisoners and civilians with TB. The coalition's press release stated, "Catastrophic growth of tuberculosis on the territory of Russia makes the problem of control over the TB epidemic very important for all the regions. At this stage, this problem ceases to be purely a medical, but becomes a social problem. At the same time, the Federal [anti-TB] Program . . . is not supported by necessary financial resources."[28]

General Vladimir Yalunin, a husky man who is the forward-looking head of the prison system of the Ministry of Justice, listened carefully. But there was no one at the meeting from the Ministry of Health. The two ministries remained in serious conflict not only over how to allocate the proposed World Bank loan but also on the most fundamental methods of TB control such as the use of DOTS.

Is Tomsk the Way to Go?

If TB was going to be controlled, the proven DOTS program would have to be added to the conventional, clunky, in-hospital Russian program, which was already short of money. Before Tomsk adopted the program, a demonstration project compared 50 patients treated with DOTS with 50 patients treated with the classical Soviet method. The cure rates were equal, but the World Health Organization's DOTS method was far cheaper and more efficient.[29] Dr. Tatiana Lyagoshina, a graduate of Tomsk medical school who works with MERLIN, collaborated with her professor, the eminent TB expert Dr. Aivar K. Strelis, on a larger study comparing patients treated in the traditional, individualized Russian way with patients treated with DOTS. Again, the cure rates were the same, but the DOTS program was two and a half times cheaper. In the prison sector, they worked with Dr. Sergei P. Mishustin, a trim, crew-cut military man who was chief doctor of Tomsk TB Colony 1. Because DOTS, although proven to be cheaper and effective, was contrary to the old Russian method. TB doctors in Tomsk had to be assured that they would not lose their jobs or pay if they switched to the World Health Organization method.

The program got an exemption from Prikaz 33, the Ministry of Health's strict order governing the way doctors must treat TB in Russia. So, in Tomsk, routine X-ray examinations for low-risk groups were eliminated, hospital beds devoted to TB were reduced by 75 percent, and the hospital stay for newly diagnosed patients was cut in half. One problem was that by Russian rules, patients were required to stay in the hospital for 2 years, even if, as is usual for drug-sensitive TB, they had been cured in 6 months or less. Staying in the hospital exposed them to reinfection with other strains of TB and made it almost impossible for them to get back to work and to support their families.

The Tomsk group adopted some ideas similar to those used in my own program in New Jersey, offering DOTS patients incentives for treatment. They set up a "day hospital" for disadvantaged patients, such as homeless people and alcoholics, where the patients could come in for the day, receive their medications, nap on comfortable cots in warm surroundings, and get two meals. A different service for working patients enabled them to come in, get their medications, and go on their way to work or home.

Nevertheless, despite its obvious success, there was resistance to the program from doctors at the regional tuberculosis hospital, who persisted in believing in long hospitalizations, with surgery on 1 in 5 patients. Rick O'Brien of the CDC says that he had lengthy discussions with surgeons about the indications for operating. He found no scientific basis for their opinions, except that, surprisingly, some seemed unaware of advances in effective medication for TB developed in the last 20 years.

Shorter, Faster, Cheaper, but Not Establishment

Tomsk TB Colony 1 takes in prisoners with TB from other prisons in the region. It is on top of a dusty hill, up an unpaved road. The entrance is difficult to find. Outside, stray dogs loiter and a number of women wait to see their men and bring them food, cigarettes, and other needs, such as a warm sweater. Some of the women are clearly mothers of the prisoners. Others look like wives or sweethearts, doing their best to be well dressed and wearing fashionably heavy makeup.

Inside, there are fierce security measures. There is an indescribable feeling of powerlessness when you must leave your passport with the guard behind a steel gate at the entry. Then you must pass through several more steel gates, each with a more ominous clang than the previous one. The thought crosses your mind increasingly, obsessively: What if the passport is not there when I want to get out? Although the buildings are middle-aged, they are neat and clean. This prison is about as good as it gets in Russia. Nevertheless, the hallways are narrow and dark, and the toilets, even for staff, are not what you would choose if you had another choice.

Tomsk TB Colony 1 has been working with Western groups for more than 5 years. Some prisoners live in large, dormitorylike rooms housing perhaps 100 or more men in double-decker bunks, not the triple-decker bunks we saw elsewhere, which limit light and air. The rooms and bunks are clean and neat. The windows let in light.

Prisoners in Tomsk TB Colony 1 are segregated by the severity of their disease. Those who have been cured of TB are assigned to jobs where they won't meet infectious prisoners. Prisoners with ordinary TB live in the wards and receive DOTS. The 200 or so prisoners who have multi-drug-resistant TB are kept in a separate area. Until recently it was a forlorn place, inhabited by incurable young men who were bereft of hope. But in September 2000, almost 50 of them started treatment with DOTS-Plus as part of a pilot program set up after extensive planning and negotiation with funders, drug manufacturers, and WHO. For the others, for the moment, there is no treatment. Some of these prisoners will probably die soon; some will finish their sentences and be released, where they can spread their untreated MDR-TB.

Although the people at the Tomsk prison are making significant progress, they have a long way to go. The guards and the nurses do not wear masks, although they are exposed to TB every day. Asked if there are negative-pressure cells for prisoners with multi-drug-resistant TB (where the air flow will direct TB bacteria away from the staff and out of the cell), Mishustin, the prison's chief physician, simply replied, "We have enough trouble feeding them." Staff at the prison are often paid in meat, in a barter system with suppliers.

Timebomb

Things seemed to be going well in Tomsk, but the situation was far worse than it appeared. As the Médecins sans Frontières project in the nearby Mariinsk TB Colony 33 showed, DOTS isn't enough. Patients who have previously been treated with some anti-TB drugs often have multi-drug-resistant TB. Giving them standard first-line drugs, even with carefully administered DOTS therapy, just encourages their TB bacteria to become resistant to more anti-TB drugs. If a DOTS program had been started 5 years ago, the explosion of multi-drug-resistant TB probably wouldn't have happened. But now the genie is out of the bottle. Only a DOTS-Plus regimen using second-line drugs would be effective now. However, DOTS-Plus requires that each patient be tested for drug sensitivity before treatment begins. Drug-sensitivity testing takes weeks and requires a sophisticated lab. When the Médecins sans Frontières program started, Khomenko's lab in Moscow was the only lab in Russia that could do these tests. Furthermore, without an absolutely reliable supply of second-line drugs, it does more harm than good to begin DOTS-Plus treatment, since breaking off the treatment fosters even more resistance.

Record keeping is another issue. Patients must be tracked; the nature and success of their treatment must be recorded, and their care must be coordinated after they leave prison. Even Professor Mikhail Perelman, who followed Dr. Alexey Priymak as the head of the Priymak institute in Moscow and Russia's top TB doctor, agrees. He told me, "The twenty-first century is the century of technology, of information." He believes that every TB patient should be recorded in a database, with information on epidemiology, the medications given, and the result of treatment. Only then will doctors have an accurate picture of the epidemic.[30]

The Tomsk project tried to set up a sophisticated computer database of patients, treatments, and results. The civilian sector used a homemade database that worked well. The prison sector used a database developed by Dr. E. Belilovsky at the Moscow Institute of Phthisiopulmonology and promoted by the Ministry of Health. Alas, it had major software flaws and data were lost, a problem that had been noticed in other regions using the database. That was a major concern because the Ministry of Health was suggesting that that database be used for implementing the proposed World Bank loan. In Tomsk, a visiting team from the Public Health Research Institute spent nearly 1 month painstakingly constructing a database from handwritten records in the prison.[31]

As it was then the only place in Russia with a coordinated anti-TB program in both the civilian and the prison sectors, Tomsk's program was reviewed by both a Russian committee (which looked at the program in the public sector[32]) and an independent international advisory committee (which looked at both the public and the prison programs[33]). As one might expect, the Russian committee regretted that the Tomsk program didn't hew more closely to traditional Russian TB treatment, and the international advisory committee regretted that the combined program didn't follow international guidelines more closely and also was worried about the sustainability of the program once the donors left. Both review committees were alarmed by the problem in Tomsk.

Despite many favorable conditions—support from an enlightened governor, assistance from international organizations, top-notch TB experts, and a reliable supply of first-line drugs—the tuberculosis problem was getting worse, not better. Although patients were receiving state-of-the-art care, only 70 percent in both the prison and the civilian sectors were being cured, because they had multi-drug-resistant TB to begin with. Of course, no one knew that at the start of the project. It was similar to the situation Médecins sans Frontières had seen in Mariinsk. When doctors used DOTS, they seemed to make matters worse, encouraging an increase in drug resistance.

The death rate from TB in Tomsk in the civilian sector was unacceptably high, almost 8 percent (the TB death rate in the United States is less than 1 percent), because so many of the cases were drug-resistant. Patients whose TB had become resistant to drugs in the prisons were dying, but they were also infecting people around them—spouses, children, neighbors, teachers, doctors and nurses, lawyers, and court officials. If these newly infected people developed active TB, it would not be ordinary, curable TB. They would have the multi-drug-resistant kind, the deadly superbug.

If this is the situation in Tomsk, with an excellent donor-supported TB-control program in both the prisons and the civilian sector, what is it like elsewhere in Russia and in the countries of the former Soviet Union? We could clearly see that the threat to Russia and the rest of the world was building. Soon, an amnesty would release 140,000 prisoners.

At the end of our visit, our team held a press conference in Moscow to report our findings. Dr. Rick O'Brien of the CDC said, "This is probably the worst situation for multi-drug-resistant tuberculosis ever documented in the world." Dr. Malgosia Grzemska of the World Health Organization said, "If we wait a year or two or more, not even the richest country in the world would be able to cope with the situation." That was in September 1998.[34]

7

The Russian Style of TB Treatment

My old friend Professor Alexander Grigorievich Khomenko lay in his coffin. He had held the highest rank in Soviet and Russian intellectual circles: academician. Khomenko had been head of the Central Tuberculosis Research Institute of the Russian Academy of Medical Sciences, the only research institute in Russia collaborating with the World Health Organization—usually respectfully referred to as the Khomenko institute. He was a world-class scientist who spoke several languages fluently and had worked for many years at the World Health Organization in Geneva to combat TB throughout the world. His had been the most powerful voice for scientific treatment of the tuberculosis epidemic that was raging in the ruins of the former Soviet Union. Now his voice was silent.

On September 27, 1999, a chilly, foggy day, 600 of Professor Khomenko's friends and colleagues crowded into the austere and monumental hall of the Central Clinical Hospital, Moscow's most distinguished medical center, set among the slim white birch trees of northwestern Moscow, for his funeral. All of them stood in respect; there were only four seats, and those were for the bereaved family. The 600 people included government ministers, distinguished professors, and representatives from the World Health Organization in Geneva, Centers for Disease Control and Prevention in Atlanta, the Public Health Research Institute in New York, and scores of other academic and clinical organizations and government ministries. Khomenko had many friends, as well as enemies.

Beneath the abstract red, gray, and black stained glass windows, the coffin rested on a raised marble slab, surrounded by flowers. At its head stood two tall brass candle stands, each with four candles. Black veiling draped the walls and the doors.

One by one, mourners came to the foot of the coffin to speak in tribute to this distinguished scientist: Professor Vladislav Yerokhin, Khomenko's deputy, soon to be his successor as head of the Central Tuberculosis Institute; Professor Alexey Priymak, former head of the Priymak institute at the Dostoyevsky Hospital, now retired, an old-school TB expert who was Khomenko's bitter rival; Professor Mikhail Perelman, who succeeded to Priymak's post after Priymak was fired, the expert favored by Russia's Ministry of Health and leader of the opposition to the WHO DOTS strategy and a passionate advocate of surgery for tuberculosis; Dr. Wieslaw Jakubowiak, the World Health Organization's soft-spoken, effective TB coordinator in Russia; Dr. Alex Goldfarb, a former Russian dissident who had left the Soviet Union more than 20 years earlier and now was the head of the Public Health Research Institute's efforts to control TB in Russia; Dr. Vitaly Litvinov, professor at the Moscow Tuberculosis Center, a leading hospital that treats the hundreds of tuberculosis patients in Moscow each year; and many, many others. It was an impressive procession of distinguished experts paying tribute to one of their own, whether they had loved him or had fought him every step of the way.

The Russian Orthodox priest, in black robes with a white cape, lit the incense in his censer and swung it as he circled the coffin three times, chanting in Old Slavonic, the ancient language of the liturgy,[1] "Blessed is our God always, now, and ever, and unto ages of ages. Amen." Smoky, fragrant incense drifted through the chill, crowded room. Two men and two women sang the hymns of the service, unaccompanied, their delicate, evocative tones floating through the marble hall.

The priest lit the lights in the candle stands, then circled the coffin again, swinging the censer. He continued his chant, "Eternal be thy memory, O our brother, who art worthy to be deemed happy and ever-memorable." "Memory eternal! Memory eternal! Memory eternal!" the choir echoed. After reading the prayer of absolution from a parchment, the priest folded it and gently slipped it into the white hand of Professor Khomenko. "O Holy God, Holy Mighty, Glory," the choir sang.

At the end, the family was left alone to say a last good-bye to his wife, Dr. Nina Khomenko, who had met Alexander when they were medical students in the terrible years at the end of World War II, and their brilliant children and grandchildren. The crowd of dignitaries moved somberly out into the damp, foggy air. They lingered on the grassy lawn outside the hall, chatting. And, because this was Russia, although many were experts in lung disease, most smoked.

What would happen now? many wondered aloud. There was a gaping hole where once there had been leadership. Both Westerners and Russians wondered who would take over Khomenko's role, not only as head of the scientifically rigorous, internationally recognized Central Tuberculosis Institute in Moscow, designated as the World Health Organization's collaborating center for Russia, but also his role as the leader and champion of effective, evidence-based, internationally approved methods of TB treatment and control. What would Khomenko's death mean for the fight against the tuberculosis epidemic surging out of Russia's huge prison Gulag? Would Yerokin, his deputy, get the job? Would Perelman and the "old Russian school" of TB treatment gain more power? Would Perelman manage to control the TB epidemic? Perelman barely gave lip service to the Western method of treatment endorsed by the World Health Organization. His heart was thought to lie elsewhere, with the traditional Russian system. If he had a say about how the rumored World Bank loan was to be spent, what would happen?

Was the epidemic going to get even worse? Was the government going to help? Was anybody going to help? Who was in charge? Whose rules would be followed? The traditional Russian way? Or the World Health Organization's highly effective program called DOTS? Khomenko had been convinced that WHO's scientifically based approach could be just as effective as the often cruel, cumbersome, expensive Russian approach, and was far cheaper. But Khomenko was dead.

What did one man's death mean for the epidemic of tuberculosis and multi-drug-resistant tuberculosis? Would Russia's epidemic continue to spread across the world?

Russia Is Different

Immediately after Khomenko's funeral, Janice Hopkins Tanne and I invited Priymak for a subdued lunch at the Golden Ring Swiss Diamond Hotel, Moscow's only five-star hotel. Removed from the chaos of the street, the Golden Ring Swiss Diamond was a cool Western-style oasis. Donald Trump would be proud of it, but it was the Swiss who had gutted an undistinguished Soviet hotel and modernized it. The building was a triumph of marble, mahogany, polished brass, and high security. The entrance and lobby were patrolled by many very large, silent men in dark suits with walkie-talkies, looking as if they had walked out of a cold war spy movie. The elevators were controlled by cards; only registered guests could reach the upper floors.

The contrast between the hotel and its surroundings, between efficient luxury and decrepit inefficiency, mirrored the state of Russia today.

Priymak drove us to the hotel in his tiny old car, and parked around the corner on a residential street. In contrast, the hotel driveway was crammed with large, dark limousines. Outside, a mess of seven or eight lanes of traffic were trying to make turns around the island at the T-shaped intersection between Smolenskaya Ulitsa and even wider Smolensky Bulvar, both major streets. Across the intersection was the Ministry of Foreign Affairs, a Stalin-era skyscraper that looked like a Gothic cathedral on drugs. Most of the cars stuck in traffic were ancient Ladas, Volgas, and other old Soviet cars, all spewing pollution into the already polluted air. People seeking a quick ride were not hailing taxis; instead, they were stopping ordinary drivers and bargaining with them. For a few rubles, usually less than a dollar—but enough to offset the high cost of gasoline—most drivers would take a detour from where they were going to drop a passenger at his or her destination.

On the little traffic island, almost bare of grass, several homeless men were already stumbling about drunk, although it was only lunchtime.

We saw more contrasts between islands of efficient luxury and the failing Russian economy. From the traffic island, a pedestrian underpass led under the 10 lanes of traffic on Smolenskaya Bulvar. It was lined with shops —shoe repair, cheap perfumes, cigarettes, vodka, and other liquor. On folding tables in the passageway, people were selling pirated CDs and computer programs. Middle-aged women were begging on the steps at the exit in front of the Ministry, where more black limousines were idling.

Yet just a hundred feet away, across a narrow street, behind a nondescript façade, was one of Moscow's best supermarkets. It had caviar, smoked fish, fresh fish, prime meats, many cheeses, fresh dairy products, crisp green vegetables—as good a selection as you'd find in New York or London, and at similar prices. Leading south from the supermarket was Arbat, an ancient pedestrian street that was part Bohemia and part tourism central—and also a sign of how decrepit Russia was. There was the ubiquitous McDonald's, cafés, bad paintings on black velvet, and tourist shops selling gold jewelry. There were also beggars, mostly needy-looking older women. Elderly grandmas were hawking diaphanous mohair shawls that they had knitted at home. Souvenir stands were selling cheap copies of Russian army watches and seemingly thousands of different traditional painted, nested dolls called matryoshka: Yeltsin on the outside, then Gorbachev, then down to Stalin or maybe a czar on the smallest inside one. Not only were there dolls representing most National Football League teams (I, of course, bought one representing the New York Giants), there was even a doll with Bill Clinton on

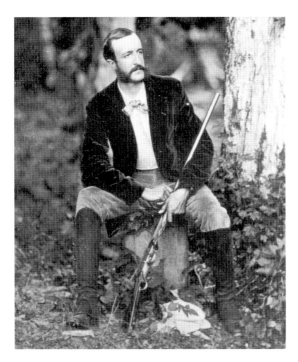

The American physician Dr. Edward Livingston Trudeau was diagnosed with tuberculosis in 1873. As his disease worsened, he moved to his beloved Adirondack Mountains in New York state to die. As this picture shows, after 3 months of fresh air and outdoor living, his health improved. (*Reprinted with permission,* © *2001, American Lung Association**)

*For more information, please visit our Web site, www.lungusa.org or call 1-800-LUNG-USA (1-800-486-4872).

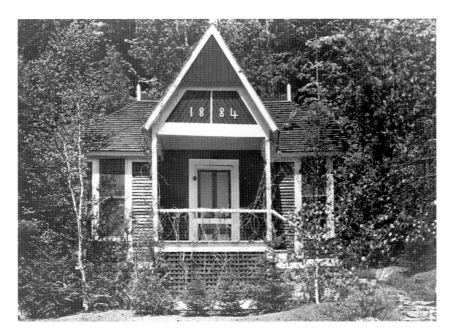

Dr. Trudeau became convinced that outdoor living and mountain air were an excellent treatment for tuberculosis, and he established the first American sanatorium at Saranac Lake in the Adirondacks. This is the first building, called "Little Red." (*Reprinted with permission* © *2001, American Lung Association*)

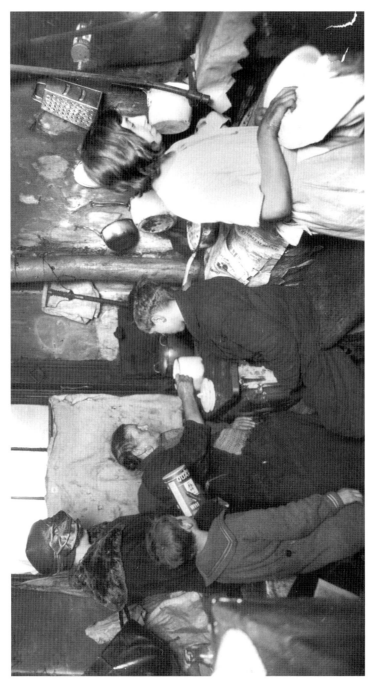

Overcrowding in bad housing spread tuberculosis during the nineteenth and early twentieth centuries. A nurse (*in hat, at left*) visits a poor family in a New York kitchen to advise on the care of family members with TB. (*Courtesy of the Chest Collection, Bellevue Hospital Archives*)

In the late nineteenth and early twentieth centuries, TB patients who could not afford to leave home for a sanatorium tried to achieve the benefits of rest and open-air living, as this woman did by sleeping in a tent on the roof of a New York tenement. The snow mimicked the mountain air of many sanatoriums. (*Courtesy of the Chest Collection, Bellevue Hospital Archives*)

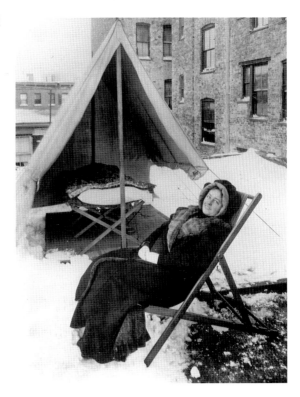

Some TB patients sought the benefits of sleeping in the open air while living in their homes. This patient's bed was raised off the floor, and she was able to sleep with her head out the window. (*Courtesy of the Chest Collection, Bellevue Hospital Archives*)

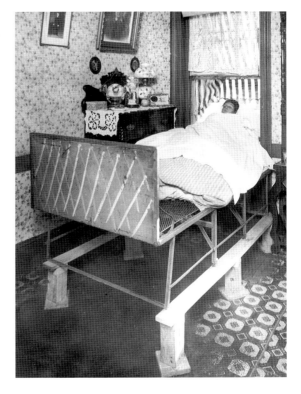

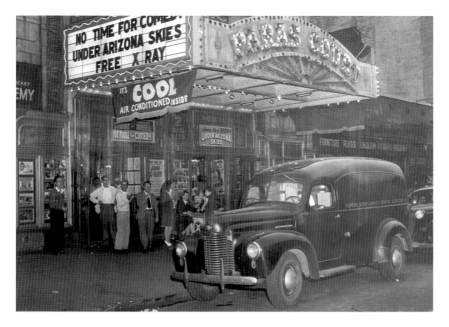

From the 1930s to the early 1970s, X-rays were widely used to detect tuberculosis in the United States. This mobile X-ray van offered free chest X-rays to moviegoers. (*Courtesy of Municipal Archives, Department of Records and Information Services, City of New York*)

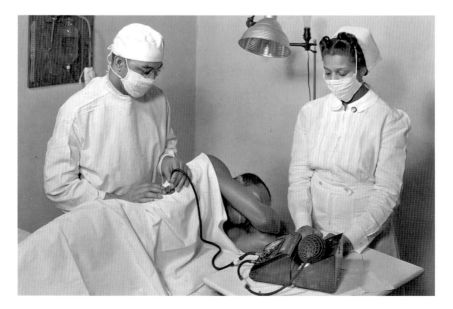

Until the 1950s, pneumothorax was used to treat patients with active tuberculosis. Air was introduced into the chest cavity by a machine, as shown here, to collapse a diseased lung. It was hoped that "resting" the lung would help it heal. Patients needed frequent "refills" of air. (*Reprinted with permission © 2001, American Lung Association*)

Estimated TB Incidence Rates, 1999 (all forms)

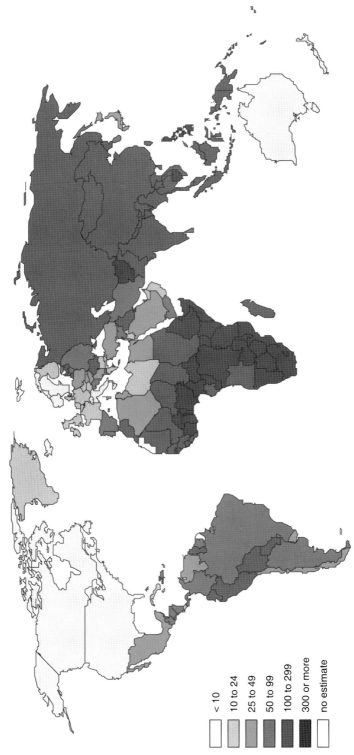

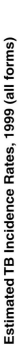

< 10
10 to 24
25 to 49
50 to 99
100 to 299
300 or more
no estimate

Estimated tuberculosis rates per 100,000 people around the world. Note the high incidence in Russia, the Far East, part of South and Central America, and Africa, where co-infection with HIV is common. (*Courtesy of the World Health Organization*)

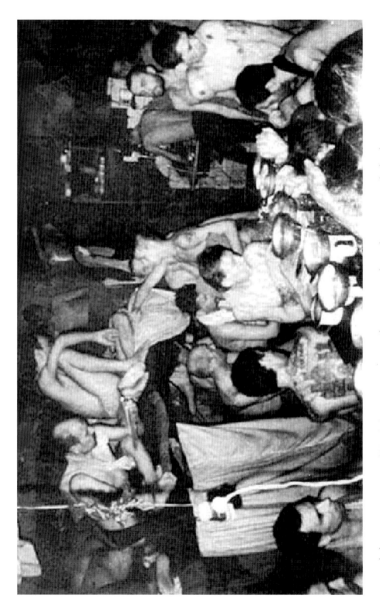

Pretrial detention centers (SIZOs) in Russia are inhumane and vastly overcrowded. They expose inmates to others with active tuberculosis, but offer little medical care. These men are awaiting trial in the notorious Matrosskaya Tishina (SIZO #1) in Moscow. SIZOs and prisons are often so overcrowded that inmates sleep in shifts. (*Courtesy of Moscow Centre for Prison Reform*)

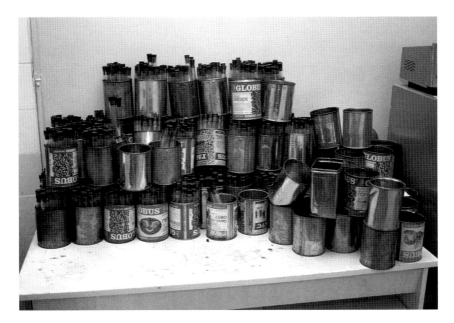

Laboratories in Russian prisons are often primitive. In the Kemerovo TB dispensary, test tubes containing infectious sputum from patients, growing on culture medium, are stored in old cans. (*Courtesy of Public Health Research Institute; photo by Sergei Gitman*)

Prison inmates in Siberia after lunch, which usually consists of a bowl of soup and a piece of black bread. (*Courtesy of Public Health Research Institute; photo by Sergei Gitman*)

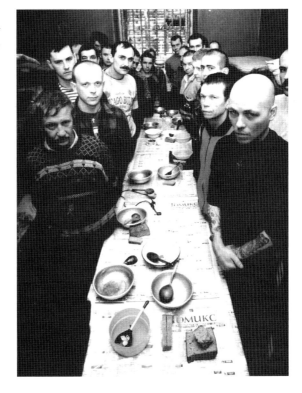

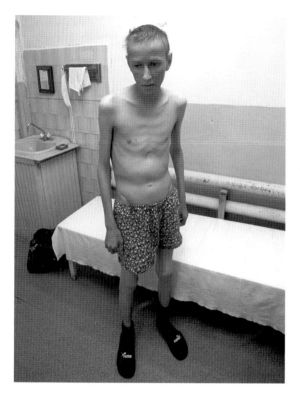

This 22-year-old young man, a second-time offender, is thought to have contracted tuberculosis while he was held in a pretrial detention center, or SIZO. His wasted appearance is typical of a patient with active TB, which causes frequent coughing, weight loss, night sweats, and fatigue. (*Courtesy of Public Health Research Institute; photo by Sergei Gitman*)

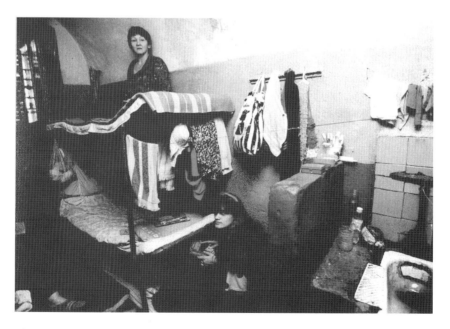

These women prisoners share a cell in Siberia. Like other Russian prisoners, they have no uniforms. Their belongings hang in plastic bags, and their wet laundry hangs on a makeshift line. (*Courtesy of Public Health Research Institute; photo by Sergei Gitman*)

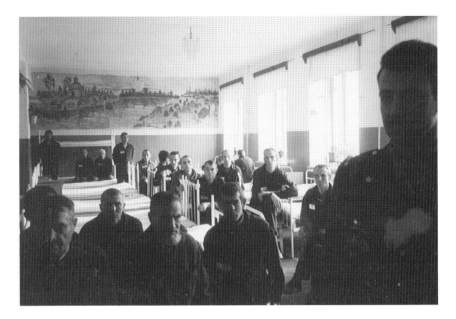

These men are held in the unit for prisoners with multi-drug-resistant TB in TB Colony 1 in Tomsk, Siberia. Note that the unit is clean and uncrowded in comparison with other prison cells, and has windows to admit sunlight and fresh air.

A prisoner with ordinary tuberculosis receives directly observed therapy from a nurse in TB Colony 1, Tomsk, Siberia. The TB colony holds prisoners with ordinary TB and multi-drug-resistant TB who are transferred from other prisons in the region.

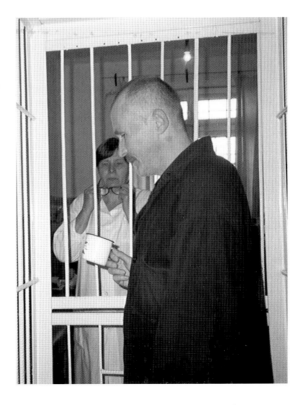

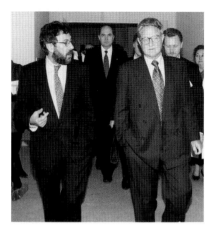

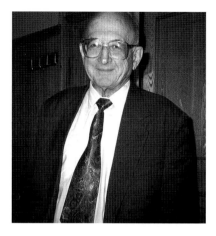

Scientist and former Russian dissident Dr. Alex Goldfarb (*left*) involved the billionaire and philanthropist George Soros (*right*) in supporting the Public Health Research Institute's effort to control tuberculosis in Russia. They are shown in the Moscow Medical Academy during a visit in 1997. (*Courtesy of Public Health Research Institute*)

Dr. Mikhail Perelman is chief phthisiologist of the Ministry of Health of the Russian Federation and is Russia's head TB doctor.

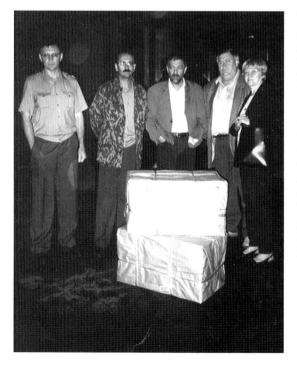

Triumph! After many difficulties, the first shipment of second-line drugs to treat multi-drug-resistant TB arrives in Tomsk. With the shipment are (*left to right*) two prison officials, Dr. Alex Goldfarb, Dr. Gennady G. Peremitin, head physician of the Tomsk Region Administration's health department, and Oksana Ponomarenko, chief program officer of the Public Health Research Institute in Moscow.

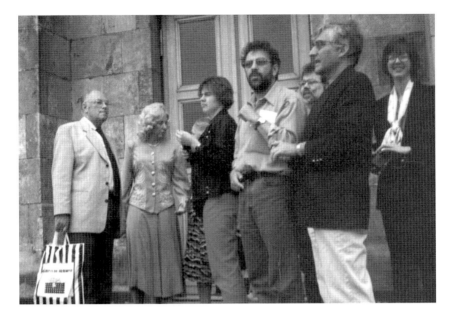

An international advisory group visited Russia in 1997 to evaluate Russian TB laboratory facilities for a possible grant from the Public Health Research Institute and the Soros Foundation. Dr. Alexey Priymak (*left*, now retired) was then Russia's leading TB physician, as chief phthisiologist of the Ministry of Health. The photo includes Dr. Priymak's assistant, our translator, Dr. Alex Goldfarb (*with beard and glasses*), Dr. Max Salfinger (*behind him*) of the Wadsworth Center, N.Y. State Department of Health, Dr. Lee B. Reichman, and Dr. Yvonne Hale of the Florida State Laboratories.

Prison doctor Natalya Vezhnina (*left*) appealed for international help to deal with the TB epidemic in TB Colony 33 in Mariinsk, Kemerovo oblast, Siberia. Dr. Malgosia Grzemska, the World Health Organization representative for TB programs in Eastern Europe (*right*), was among the experts who made an inspection visit. Note the protective respirator (mask) around Dr. Grzemska's neck, ready to be put on when she enters the prison. Like almost all Russian prison personnel, Dr. Vezhnina has no respirator.

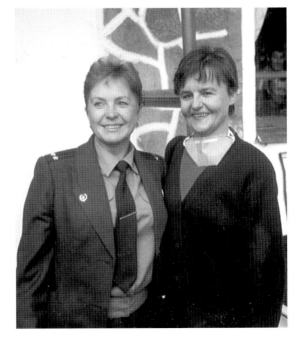

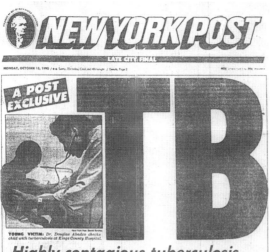

In the late 1980s and early 1990s, New York City and the nation suffered an epidemic of tuberculosis after funding to control the disease was cut. The story was headline news in the local and national press. (*Courtesy of New York Post*)

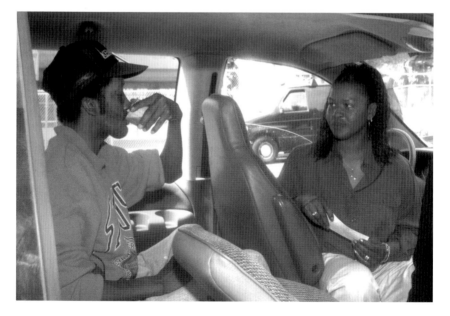

Directly observed therapy (DOT) means making sure that each patient takes appropriate medication to cure tuberculosis. Field worker Rebecca Stevens from the N.J. Medical School National Tuberculosis Center delivers DOT to one of her patients in her van on the street in Newark, NJ. (*Courtesy of New Jersey Medical School, National Tuberculosis Center, Newark, NJ*)

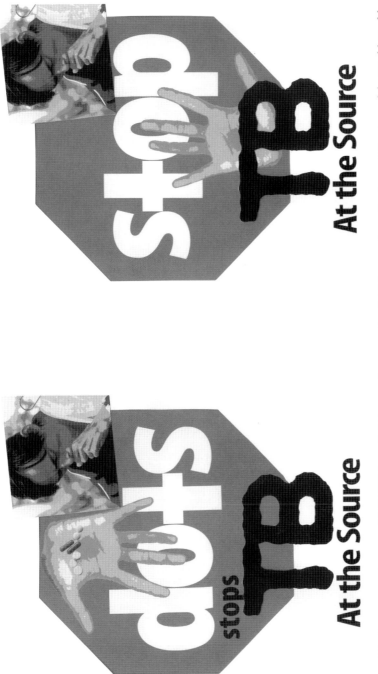

The World Health Organization's powerful DOTS logo (*left*) is merely a stop sign (*right*) turned upside down. (*Courtesy of the World Health Organization, Global Tuberculosis Programme, Stop TB at the Source: 1995 Annual Report on the Tuberculosis Epidemic, Geneva, Switzerland*)

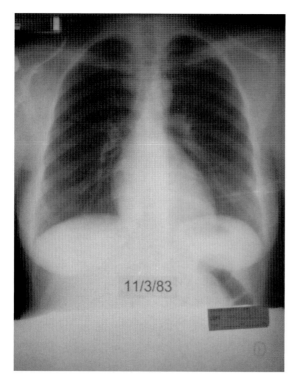

X-ray of a 40-year-old nurse with a positive skin test for TB who had received BCG vaccination in the past. She refused treatment because of her previous BCG vaccination, although her physicians thought she had latent tuberculosis infection. (*Courtesy of University Hospital, Department of Radiology, New Jersey Medical School*)

11/3/83

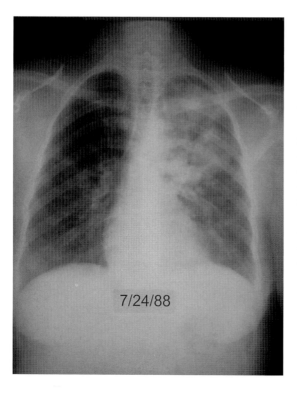

Five years later, the nurse had extensive tuberculosis involving the upper part of her left lung (the new white area in her left lung, which appears on the right in the X-ray). She had multi-drug-resistant TB and was cured after 2½ years of intensive, daily, directly observed therapy with second-line drugs. (*Courtesy of University Hospital, Department of Radiology, New Jersey Medical School*)

7/24/88

	1	W101
	2	W106
	3	W186
	4	W206
	5	W214
	6	W217
	7	W148
	8	W15
	9	W
	10	W1
	11	W12
	12	W4
	13	C
	14	U
	15	AH
	16	AB
	17	P
	18	N
	19	N3

DNA fingerprinting reveals whether TB strains are similar or unrelated. Lanes 1–12 (numbered from top down at the next-to-last column at the right) are members of the notorious strain W family. Subgroups of the W family are noted in the far right column (W101, W106, etc.). Strain W caused many cases in the New York City epidemic. Note the similarity of the bar patterns. (Lanes 1 and 2 are from Singapore; 3–7 from Russia; 8 from Kenya; 9–11 from New York City; 12 from New Jersey.) Lanes 13–19 show the range of different DNA fingerprint patterns found in New York City, except for lane 14, which is from New Jersey. (*Courtesy of Marcel Dekker, Inc., New York, from Tuberculosis: A Comprehensive International Approach, 2d ed., 2000, Courtesy of Public Health Research Institute, Dr. Barry Kreiswirth*)

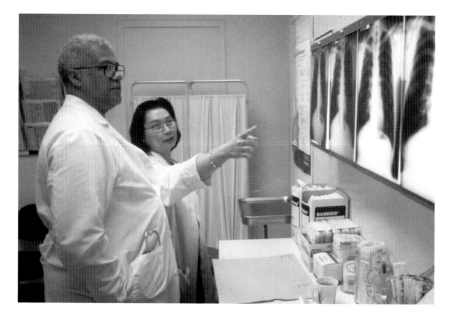

At the New Jersey Medical School National Tuberculosis Center in Newark, Drs. Reynard McDonald and Bonita Mangura examine chest X-rays of patients recently treated and cured of TB at Newark's University Hospital. (*Courtesy of New Jersey Medical School*)

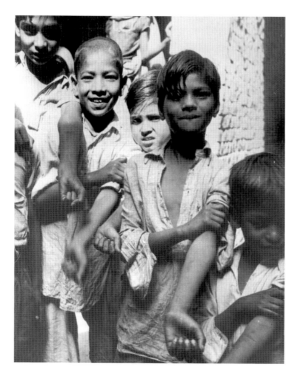

After World War II, BCG vaccine—which has variable effectiveness—was used by the World Health Organization in an attempt to protect children against TB. The vaccine, developed by French scientists, has been widely used since the 1920s. These youngsters in Delhi in 1964 show off their injection scars. Scientists hope to develop a truly effective vaccine in the next few decades. (*Courtesy of the American Lung Association and the World Health Organization*)

the outside, then Hillary, Monica, and finally a cigar on the inside. Three people were selling kittens.

When Priymak, Janice, and I reached the elegant, spacious restaurant on the second floor of the Golden Ring Swiss Diamond Hotel, with its multilingual service, fine linens, and good silver, we found that we were the only diners. We were very polite with Priymak. In this upholstered green haven, we did not mention my own visit 2 years previously with the team that was evaluating his lab, nor his outburst at the meeting of the Gore-Chernomyrdin commission, 2 months later, which had directly led to his firing.

At the hotel, we ordered our lunch: appetizers of smoked salmon and sturgeon, a salad, and baked fish. I ordered a beer, but Priymak declined: "I'm driving," he said. Speaking through an interpreter, Priymak said that he was happily retired. He was lively and friendly. His dark blue eyes sparkled in his ruddy face as he told us that he was living on a lake near Moscow where he could indulge his passion for sailing his small boat. In the United States, I thought, such a distinguished physician would most likely be living in a Florida condo and sailing something much larger than Alexey's small sailboat. Being a doctor is neither highly respected nor well paid in Russia.

Like many tuberculosis experts, Priymak entered the field because the disease had altered his life. "My father was in the military. He got TB," he said. "I was about 11 when he first became ill. I observed, and I decided to become a doctor. He died of it some years later. Everyone from my father's side of the family was ill with TB. Only I and my son and my two grandchildren are well."

He was noticeably more wary when we talked about Russia's current tuberculosis problem, saying that journalists had misinterpreted his views in the past, and Janice, a journalist, was here with us at lunch. We assured him that although we might not always agree with him, we would present his views fairly.

"Russia is different and TB is different in Russia," Priymak said. "You have to know our history. In World War I, 1914 to 1918, we lost 1 million people at the front. But meanwhile, 2 million people died of tuberculosis." The World War I epidemic prompted the Soviet state to set up a national system to fight tuberculosis. There was a special tuberculosis department in the Ministry of Health, separate from the regular health-care system. Every region had a tuberculosis institute for treatment of patients, for research, and for training phthisiologists (TB specialists).

"In World War II," Priymak continued, "Russia was thrown back. We started again from zero." During that war, which Russians call "the Great

Patriotic War," probably 26 million civilians died in the warfare, or of disease and famine at home. The country was devastated. Tuberculosis soared. In the late 1940s, after World War II ended, the first drugs for TB became available to Russian doctors. They included streptomycin, the drug that saved Khomenko's life as a young medical student, and later isoniazid.

The Old Way

Priymak explained how, after World War II, the Soviet Union rebuilt its massive, centralized system to fight TB. About 20 tuberculosis research institutes were established, six of them in Russia and the others in other states of the former Soviet Union. Cut off from scientific developments in the rest of the world, Soviet doctors developed their own approaches to treatment, which understandably, without scientific exchange and communication, differed from international standards. In addition, there were (and still are) completely separate hospitals and health systems for people who work in the railroad and shipping industries.

In the early 1990s, the breakup of the Soviet Union and the economic collapse that followed threw the system into disarray. Medical staff weren't paid for months, the drug supply was erratic, and X-ray machines broke down, or X-ray film wasn't available. Isolated and unaware of scientific developments in the international TB community, Soviet doctors clung to their old views of tuberculosis and how it should be treated. Many Russian doctors still hold these views today and are confused by the conflicting messages from the World Health Organization and from their own Russian experts.

To this day, many Russian scientists believe that directly or indirectly, tuberculosis affects every part of the patient's body, not just the lungs. Therefore, the disease varies from patient to patient, and treatment must be tailored to each patient, taking into consideration the state of the patient's liver and gastrointestinal tract (which might be affected by side effects of medications), and whether the patient's body metabolizes drugs slowly or quickly. Therefore, doses can be raised or lowered, drugs added or subtracted from the regimen, as the doctor thinks best. The drugs may be given orally as pills, intravenously, or, in procedures never done in the West, injected directly into the TB cavity in the lungs through a bronchoscope (a long tube inserted down the windpipe into the lung) or through the chest wall right into the lungs by a needle. TB drugs are often supplemented by "pathogenetic therapy," a sort of support therapy that may include anti-inflammatory drugs, agents thought to improve the immune system, vitamins, detoxifying agents, drugs to improve the circulation, liver tonics, exposure of blood to ultraviolet rays (the blood is removed from the patient, exposed to ultraviolet light, and then returned to the patient by transfusion), and many other treatments, as the doctor decides. Such scientifically unproven therapy is virtually never done in other countries.[2]

It seems obvious to me that by individualizing treatment, the Russian method encourages the development of drug resistance and multi-drug resistance, which usually occurs when the patient doesn't get the full course of effective antibiotics, when the drugs are given at too low a dose, or when some drugs are taken alone, instead of in the complete regimen of several effective drugs.

A major, global breakthrough in TB treatment occurred in 1986, when the World Health Organization endorsed the DOTS treatment strategy originally developed by Karel Styblo of the International Union Against Tuberculosis and Lung Disease and first proven effective in Africa among people who were poor and illiterate. In 1995, The term DOTS was adopted as a brand name by WHO with the assistance of a high-powered Washington public relations firm because, when it is set in lower case type and reversed, "dots" turns into "stop." So the tag line became "Stop TB, use DOTS." DOTS uses a standardized combination of drugs that has been shown to cure most patients with ordinary TB, and therefore usually prevents the development of multi-drug-resistant TB as well.

DOTS has now been endorsed by 128 countries, but emphatically not by Russia. Priymak did not believe in DOTS. He thought it was suitable only for Third World countries and called it "soup-kitchen medicine." He considered it inappropriate for Russia, with its sophisticated medical system.

In the USSR, the effort to prevent TB began at birth. Starting in 1925, soon after the BCG vaccine was developed, all babies in the republics of the Soviet Union had to be vaccinated within days of their birth. They still do. In Russia today, more than 90 percent of babies receive a BCG shot, usually before they leave the hospital or maternity home with their mothers. Perhaps 60 percent get another shot at the age of 6 or 7, and about 40 percent get another at age 14 or 15. Yet another dose of vaccine may be given at age 28, particularly to those whose skin test is negative.[3] The cost is substantial: Laboratories must produce and package the vaccine, nurses and doctors must administer it, and clerks must keep voluminous records. Even knowledgeable doctors who believe that BCG may have some benefit in protecting infants and young children against serious TB disease agree that multiple vaccinations over a lifetime are not beneficial. Nevertheless, the Russians have persisted in believing that BCG can protect the whole population from TB, despite the well-documented fact that Russia has a growing TB epidemic among its citizens, most of whom have been vaccinated several times.

The Russians also believe that TB cases can be found by massive screening efforts. In the old system, before the collapse of communism in 1991, all Soviet citizens were required to have a chest X-ray every other year, a method the West abandoned in the 1960s. People in special categories, such as those who worked in public catering facilities, salespeople in shops, workers in day-care centers, and those who were chronically ill, had to have a chest X-ray each year. Everyone had to produce a normal X-ray in order to get a job.[4] After the Chernobyl nuclear accident in 1986, people became reluctant to undergo regular X-rays for fear of the radiation.

Russian establishment experts would like to see this system restored or enhanced. They argue that X-rays pick up TB at the earliest stage. More often than not, however, a suspicious sign on an X-ray is an old, healed scar or some other noninfectious disease rather than active TB. Frequent, periodic X-rays as practiced in Russia (and too often, I regret to say, in the West) are in fact a woefully inefficient and expensive way to pick up previously undiagnosed TB, and they expose people to unnecessary radiation. If a person has no TB on the day the X-ray is taken, the X-ray promotes a false sense of security, even if symptoms develop later. But the disease may start soon *after* the X-ray is taken, and, unless symptoms appear (which is the usual way of diagnosing TB), it may go undetected. It is more efficient and cost-effective to screen only patients with suspicious clinical findings such as a cough, wasting, and weight loss or people who have been exposed to a person with infectious TB. Targeted screening, where only patients who exhibit symptoms are given X-rays, is more effective and far cheaper than taking an X-ray of everybody, whether she or he has symptoms or not. But even with symptomatic patients, most Western TB experts believe that diagnosis must be made by acid-fast smear (examination of sputum under a microscope) and confirmed by the "gold standard" of bacteriologic culture of the sputum, which will show whether TB bacteria can be grown from the sputum.

Despite general X-ray screening, tuberculosis often went undiagnosed in Russia. Because the TB service and the general health service were separate, general physicians were less likely to suspect TB in their patients, leading to correct diagnosis at a much later stage of the disease.[5] Furthermore, Russian public health law required that TB patients be confined in a hospital for 1 to 2 years, even if they were cured before their term was completed. Thus many people tried to avoid being diagnosed, even those with severe symptoms who were infecting others. After a year or two in the hospital, a TB patient would almost certainly have lost his or her job. Obviously, families of TB patients suffered economically.

Dr. Tatiana Lyagoshina, a Russian TB clinician who works with the British medical-aid group MERLIN in Tomsk, Siberia, has written, "To fall ill with tuberculosis in Russia still causes pain, shame, and hopelessness, because the system works against tuberculosis patients, despite all the governmental declarations about equal care and respect for any patient. For example, if you are a teacher, medic, or cook and ever had tuberculosis registered by the dispensary, your chances of returning to your profession are between very slight and . . . nil. The history of extra-long multiple treatment courses, the bad reputation and negative impact on personal life makes people fear the disease and those who bear it. It will take years and years to overcome the fear of tuberculosis in the society."[6]

Before the collapse of the Soviet Union, everyone diagnosed with TB was hospitalized for a year or more in special TB hospitals, and then was often sent to a health resort, rather like the old sanatoriums in the United States. Today, Russian TB experts struggle to maintain this system, even though they often run short of drugs and supplies such as X-ray film.

These draconian measures might have helped patients who lived desperate lives, such as the homeless or drug-addicted, but they were unnecessary for many patients, and they did little to reduce the risk of transmission of TB to the community. However, Priymak did give two valid reasons why the Russians continued to treat TB on an inpatient basis: the vast Russian distances and the thousands of tiny villages. Since most of the younger people had moved to the cities, many villages in Russia had only three or four elderly inhabitants, with the next village perhaps 300 miles away. Some villages could be reached only in winter, when the swamps had frozen over. Others could be reached only in warm weather, when the snow had melted. Thus, people in these remote settlements were often very ill before they were diagnosed and required immediate hospitalization. Furthermore, if they were sent back home for outpatient treatment, there would be no one to bring them their medicines or check their condition.

In the Russian system, follow-up treatment continued for at least several years, and usually for a lifetime. Some patients, considered "chronics," received 3 months of the TB medicine isoniazid every spring and fall, which were thought by some Russian doctors to be times of low immunity and susceptibility to reactivation of TB. We found this to be one of the strangest of all Russian TB treatments. There was absolutely no scientific justification for this practice. It not only led to unnecessary expenditures for drugs and follow-up, but it also caused unnecessary drug side effects.

In Russia, a TB patient was not considered cured until there were no bacteria in the sputum, there was absolutely no remaining X-ray evidence of disease, and the patient had been socially rehabilitated. In contrast, Western experts considered a patient cured merely after he or she had completed drug treatment and produced negative sputum. Healed TB scars were a reason the Russians relied on surgery. Since a clear X-ray was required for a definition of cure, people in jobs dealing with the public, such as doctors, nurses, or teachers, could not go back to work unless they were positively declared cured of tuberculosis. According to the Russian idea of what constituted a cure, this meant that they could not have any healed scars. Such scars, which are a natural response to the healing process, are seen in *the vast majority* of cured TB patients and are harmless. Repeated studies have shown that in an adequately treated patient, scars are unrelated to *any* risk of relapse. But, as you might expect, many Russians with these healed scars still chose surgery, or even asked for it, because that was the only way to get rid of the scars on their chest X-rays so that they could go back to work.[7]

The Russian Resurgence

The old Soviet system was clunky, expensive, old-fashioned, overorganized, and intrusive, and it had many unnecessary components, but it did seem to work. Effective medicines and good organization—the essential parts of any successful TB control program—led to a sharp drop in the reported tuberculosis rate. At our lunch meeting, Priymak explained, "During Soviet times [before 1991], social security was better. Salaries were low, but apartment rents were cheap. Starting from birth, a person felt socially secure and was educated. In the 1970s, TB dropped by 4 percent per year. Then increased surgical treatment began around 1980. There were about 20,000 operations for TB every year. We had high-quality diagnosis with fluorography [a type of X-ray procedure]. 1986 was the peak of fighting TB. We had 100,000 beds in hospitals, 30,000 beds in health centers, and 10,000 TB specialists. The TB rate was 30 per 100,000 people. In children it was 4 or 5 per 100,000. The death rate was 10 per 100,000."

In the United States in the same year, the TB rate was only 9.4 per 100,000, and almost all patients were treated as outpatients. Today there are probably fewer than 300 TB beds in the entire United States, mostly for the rare TB patients who need long-term care or the small number who are being confined because they refuse to comply with treatment and are thus a threat to public health. In addition, hospitals like mine have respiratory isolation units. These are not specifically TB beds, but rooms where doctors can iso-late patients with any dangerous airborne infection.[8] Where I work, in Newark's University Hospital, a 500-bed facility which houses a national tuberculosis center, we have 49 rooms that can be used as respiratory isola-tion rooms (or for other purposes), but we rarely have more than two or three TB patients in the hospital at any one time.

By the 1970s, most TB sanatoriums in the United States had been closed. American politicians saw the continuing success in the fight against TB and thought that there was no need to finish the job. They began cutting funds, leading directly to a national outbreak of tuberculosis and the headline-making New York City epidemic in the late 1980s and early 1990s.

In an eerily similar way, the same thing happened in the Soviet Union in the late 1980s. Priymak said, "With a sharp drop in TB rates, people said we didn't need a special TB organization." Priymak could see the storm com-ing. Like a good sailor, he charted its possible courses. "In 1986 I created a TB database. My reasoning was that if we prepared the Russian program to fight tuberculosis effectively, we would have a sharp drop in tuberculosis. If we had no effective program, we would see a sharp increase. TB rates would increase to 70 or 80 per 100,000 people, with death rates from TB of 30 per 100,000, and children infected at the rate of 20 per 100,000." Priymak was very prescient about the looming epidemic: TB rates in Russia rose from 34 per 100,000 in 1991 to 82 per 100,000 in 1997, just as he had predicted,[9] and are even higher now. Recently, the rate rose again to 85 per 100,000.[10]

It is difficult to measure the extent of the resurgence of TB in Russia because there is no way of knowing what the TB rates under the old Soviet system really were. Russian TB experts agree that the old system did keep TB rates relatively low, but they also admit that the system lied to its own doctors and to international authorities that collect TB statistics, such as the World Health Organization. In an interview at his hospital in Tomsk, Siberia, Professor Aivar Karlovich Strelis, dean of the medical faculty and head of the department of phthisiology at the Siberian Medical University, one of the most important medical schools in Russia, said, "In Soviet times, TB rates were not spoken of. They were kept secret. You could speak of it only to [professional] societies. . . . Our work was cut off from the rest of the world. Although there were many TB experts [working] at a very good scientific level, the data were not reliable. During the last 9 years [since the breakup of the Soviet Union], everything has changed."[11] In a September 1997 article in the newsweekly *Itogi*, journalist Masha Gessen documented the same story, interviewing many experts who wanted to remain anonymous but who attested that the old Soviet numbers were lies.[12]

Even Perelman, Priymak's successor and today the most important TB expert in Russia, later told us, "All statistics on tuberculosis were a state secret until 1992. We didn't know what was happening. We didn't give the statistics to WHO. We were in the dark. We have been working in an open society only for 7 or 8 years."[13]

The tough times that followed the breakup of the Soviet Union in 1991 nurtured tuberculosis. Malnutrition, unemployment, and refugees fueled the fire of tuberculosis and other diseases. People were desperately fleeing from the war-ravaged northern Caucasus, Armenia, and Chechnya, crowding into cities, living with friends or relatives, sometimes begging in the streets. Many of them turned up in Moscow's TB hospitals, brought by their relatives. Added to this was the growing number of prisoners, which, Priymak pointed out, could be considered another migrant population. They were moved from where they had been arrested to the SIZOs, then they were moved back and forth to court, then they were moved to the prisons. When they were released, some of them moved to Moscow and other large cities, and many lived on the streets, in the metro system, in the busy railroad stations, and in street underpasses. Priymak described the current situation to us. "Fifty percent of the population lives below the poverty level. By age 14, 50 percent of the population are infected with TB. In adults, 60 to 70 percent are infected, 80 percent by the time people are in their 60s or 70s."

Priymak also gave us his grim view of Russia's future: "AIDS will impact TB. We've detected approximately 10,000 cases of AIDS so far [the number was estimated in July 2001 to have grown to 750,000], but there are many more cases not diagnosed. The future is very unpleasant. One should not hope for better times. In 3 to 5 years we'll see the spread of extra-pulmonary TB [TB affecting other parts of the body, like our 'weird TB' in New Jersey at the start of the AIDS epidemic]. More often TB will be accompanied by other diseases. . . . Doctors should be ready."

Of course, the most troubling aspect of the situation was that it nurtured the rise of multi-drug-resistant tuberculosis. The old, rigid Soviet TB system had at least had good organization and a reliable supply of drugs. When the Soviet Union collapsed, there was no longer a reliable supply of drugs, and the population was weakened by malnutrition, alcoholism, and unemployment. The prisons were overcrowded and often unable to treat TB patients. Doctors gave TB patients whatever drugs were available, which was exactly the way to create multi-drug-resistant tuberculosis. Multi-drug-resistant TB was being propagated and was rapidly spilling out of prisons into the general population.

Many international TB experts—and some Russian ones—agreed with Goldfarb, the head of the Public Health Research Institute program in Russia, who felt that the Russian TB establishment was overdue for a complete restructuring. According to Goldfarb, "Russia needs to go through a transformation like that of the West in the 1950s. The sanatoriums, the specialist TB hospitals, the isolation of patients—all that needs to be dismantled and replaced by a modern, broad-based system. The old system was expensive and inefficient. There's a huge national network of specialist institutions and dispensaries. TB patients were supposed to be confined. There was no standard treatment. When you look at it, it's like moving backward in a time machine. By 4 or 5 years ago, the system wasn't functioning any more. There was no X-ray film. The mandatory screening wasn't working any more. Patients didn't want to go to hospital. But the network was still there. The establishment resisted dismantling and setting up a community-based system."

But specific and expensive hospital systems have a way of persisting. Even in the United States it took 25 years after the effective TB drugs were introduced to close sanatoriums in my state.

Similarly, the old Russian system still prevailed and was hard to dismantle, for very good economic reasons. As British prison expert Vivien Stern wrote, "In Russia there are 84,000 pulmonary hospital beds and 10,000 lung physicians. The payment system is an incentive to put patients in hospital and operate on them. The pay of hard-pressed Russian medical staff is based on the number of filled beds and the number of operations completed. A switch to a regime requiring personnel with fewer qualifications to administer drugs to people living at home and coming to the dispensary every day would mean redeployment or redundancy [unemployment] for many. It would call for a massive reform of the public health system and a switch from hospital to primary health care."[14]

Khomenko had felt that moving to the DOTS program was the way to treat TB patients more efficiently and economically, given Russia's economic plight. As Shalala, then U.S. Secretary of Health and Human Service, said at the Gore-Chernomyrdin commission meeting, DOTS programs could simply be added to the existing Russian system. But the real crunch is that since the World Bank would like to lend Russia $100 million for TB control, what conditions will the World Bank place on the procedures used by Russia's health officials and doctors?

Rebuilding the Old System

A few days after our lunch with Priymak, Janice and I met his colleague and successor, Perelman, and his deputy, Professor Irine Bogadelnikova.[15] We wanted to hear their opinions about what should be done with the Russian system for treating TB. Russian and World Bank officials will have to agree on how the loan is to be used, with advice from both Russian and international experts on TB. Perelman was the Ministry of Health's official TB expert.

We took them to dinner at the sophisticated restaurant on top of our hotel, on the twenty-third floor. Everything was upholstered, carpeted, and luxurious, with chandeliers and mirrors. The setting was perfect, except for enthusiastic musicians, who had to be quieted so that we could talk, And again, we were the only diners in the entire restaurant. As dusk fell, the lights of Moscow came up around us. At that height and with the heavy drapes and thick windows, we were insulated for a time from the problems of the day. All we could see of the city were the lights.

Although we were all polite and cordial, we were wary, like prizefighters circling each other. The politics of TB in Russia are as complicated as public health politics anywhere, and then some. On the broader political scene, the Communist party endorsed "national values," which usually meant restoring the monolithic systems prevalent in the Soviet Union, and opposed Western ideas that they felt were being foisted on them by patronizing foreigners. Russia, after all, was still a major power with an arsenal of nuclear missiles.

Like so many Russian TB experts, Perelman was a thoracic surgeon who specialized in surgery for tuberculosis. He reminded us that he had published a comprehensive paper on surgery for TB in the *World Journal of Surgery* a few years earlier.[16] He is a big, jovial, forceful, balding man in his mid-seventies, a voluble and enthusiastic talker—so enthusiastic that our interpreter had little time for eating. Bogadelnikova, a pretty, stylish, smart, and organized blonde in her forties, is in charge of teaching medical students at the Priymak institute at the Dostoyevsky Hospital. She said little as Perelman strongly presented his views.

Perelman made it clear to us that his first priorities were investments in education, both medical and public, and in information technology to monitor patient treatment and results and to detect drug resistance. We couldn't argue with that. When it came to diagnosis and treatment, however, he argued forcefully for rebuilding the former Soviet system, with some modifications. He acknowledged that there was no longer enough money to

X-ray the entire population. "We have to change tactics," he said, "and X-ray only the population at risk. This differs in different regions from year to year, depending on economic conditions." He maintained that routine screening should be done for medical people who work with tuberculosis patients; the homeless and alcoholics and those who work with them; people with problems such as diabetes, immunodeficiency, or cancer; and the elderly.

In children, Perelman said, the tuberculin skin test was the only way to detect tuberculosis. He admitted that the BCG vaccine did not offer 100 percent protection against TB, but he insisted that it did protect young children from TB meningitis. He maintained that Russian doctors could distinguish between a positive skin test produced by BCG and a positive skin test caused by tuberculosis infection. He said it was a matter of the size of the red bump and how long ago the child received BCG. To me that sounded as accurate as reading tea leaves.

The World Health Organization, whose approach might well be adopted by the World Bank in the upcoming loan negotiations, advocated abandoning X-ray diagnosis altogether in favor of diagnosis by acid-fast smear (microscopic examination of the sputum) as part of the DOTS strategy. This was a relatively simple method that can be used even in primitive conditions, if necessary.

Perelman didn't have much faith in sputum testing anyway, believing that X-rays were much better for early detection of TB. He argued for replacing Russia's old X-ray equipment with new digital X-ray technology. "The radiation is much, much less. The quality of the image is much better. Equipment by Philips or Toshiba costs $400,000 to $500,000 (per unit). Similar equipment is produced in Russia; it's only a little bit less sophisticated, but it costs only $75,000."

Nevertheless, Perelman agreed, "The main method of treatment is drugs. That goes without saying." When he talked about problems with DOTS, the "gold standard" recommended by the World Health Organization and international TB experts, he gave us an important clue to understanding the Russian resistance to this extraordinarily effective treatment method. It had to do with the word "standard." "Standard" had been translated into Russian as "primitive" or "simplified" or "basic," he explained. No Russian patient would want to have the simplest, most basic treatment when he or she could get sophisticated treatment, the real stuff that worked. So there was great resistance to DOTS in Russia that Perelman asserted was purely semantic in origin.

Russian doctors also continued to believe in individualizing treatment, adjusting drugs and dosages. "The patient must be treated, not the disease,"

Perelman said. "We have a joke: Standards are very good if the doctor has no time to think." He noted with scorn that in Africa DOTS is given not by doctors but by social workers or outreach workers. Indeed, that was the way we did it at the New Jersey Medical School National Tuberculosis Center, after diagnosis and with follow-up by doctors. It worked. We had an astounding 98 percent cure rate in a group of high-risk patients with major social problems like alcoholism, drug addiction, homelessness, and AIDS. But in Perelman's opinion, DOTS was a method for Third World countries, not for a sophisticated industrialized country like Russia. He was sure that Russian patients, as well as Russian doctors, would never accept DOTS. He told us that social workers in Russia did not do this sort of work. "I doubt we could install such a system quickly," he said. "It's a social, not a medical system. The mentality of the people here is different. It's difficult to make people swallow pills."

Perelman continued to emphasize how different TB is in Russia. He insisted that Russian patients are sicker than those in the United States. "They have many accompanying diseases, and it is difficult to select the appropriate therapy because of the side effects of therapy," he said. That led to doctors individualizing treatment, by changing antibiotics, which led to multi-drug resistance.

Russia had a category of TB patients called "chronics"; we did not. Our patients—and theirs—felt better after about a month of treatment. If our patients had stopped taking the pills before the course of therapy was completed, they might have become "chronics," but our outreach workers made sure they completed their treatment. Perelman admitted that many Russian "chronic" TB patients were alcoholics or homeless. It was difficult to get them to cooperate with treatment. "DOTS couldn't be implemented here. It's a social problem," he said again, as if our TB patients in New Jersey did not have similar problems. He did not seem to appreciate an important difference in our approaches to drug treatment. In Russia, the patient must go to the TB dispensary every day to get his or her medication, taking time off from work, traveling a long, inconvenient distance, finding somebody to watch the children. In Newark, we try to be as positive and convenient for the patients as possible. We go to the patients—at home, at a bar, at a day-care center, at the railroad station, at the crack dens where people do drugs, on a street corner, or wherever we can find them. We try to make treatment easy for patients, and in return, we offer an incentive: We may give them bus coupons, cans of a nutritional supplement, even coupons to fast-food restaurants.

Perhaps most importantly, Russia lacked an adequate, reliable supply of drugs. "Treatment requires medicines," Perelman said. "We don't have enough medicines. The state budget tries, but it's not enough. Moscow has enough medicines, but the other regions don't. WHO and other donor organizations provide assistance to some regions."

Until now, Russian doctors had never needed to consider the cost of treatment. During the Soviet period, cost was not a concern, and that culture still lingered. Perelman explained it thus: "Before, doctors didn't need to count the cost. Every time I visit the United States, to an institution like Memorial Sloan-Kettering [a leading cancer center in New York], I look with great surprise at how doctors discuss finances. In Russia, it's not polite, not decent to talk money. You talk health, life, not money." DOTS might well be cheaper than the old way, but it was going to be an uphill battle to get the Russian TB establishment to accept it, partly because doctors felt it unseemly to talk about money.

While we were on the subject of money, I raised the issue of the proposed World Bank loan, which even at that time (September 1999) seemed to hinge on a change in Russian attitudes. Perelman was confident that 99 percent of Russian doctors agreed with his method of treating tuberculosis: diagnosis by X-ray rather than sputum smear, lengthy hospitalization, and often surgery. Only 1 percent would be interested in obtaining money from the World Bank if it meant a change in practice, he claimed.

"Let me talk absolutely frankly, because it is necessary," he said. "I think we would say yes to the World Bank, to get the money, but then we would do our own thing. The World Bank doesn't define the method of treatment. It only gives money."

8
Fingerprinting the Bacteria

In March 2000, the New York City Department of Health sent a culture of tuberculosis bacteria from a recently diagnosed patient to Dr. Barry Kreiswirth's lab at the Public Health Research Institute. They asked Kreiswirth, a molecular biologist, to do DNA fingerprinting of the bacteria. The patient had active, infectious tuberculosis and had coughed up a sample of sputum. Only living TB bacteria can be fingerprinted. At present, there is no way of retrieving and fingerprinting TB bacteria that may be lying latent in someone's body. Kreiswirth's lab is one of seven centers designated by the Centers for Disease Control and Prevention (CDC) to do DNA fingerprinting of TB bacteria. Since 1992 it has been using a sophisticated computer program to catalog and compare the DNA fingerprints of tuberculosis strains. The fingerprint technique involves looking for common markers in strains of TB bacteria from different patients. It can detect outbreaks, show where TB is being transmitted in a given population, and reveal how drug-resistant strains of TB are spreading in hospitals, cities, countries, continents, and across oceans.

Kreiswirth's lab has the world's largest collection of DNA fingerprints of TB bacteria. Its computerized database holds 12,000 strains from around the globe, including 1500 from TB patients in the civilian and prison population in Russia. About 8000 strains in the database, while they are not identical, share some genetic similarities, which provide clues to where the TB bacteria came from, the pattern of their spread, and whether they are multidrug-resistant. Each sample is coded, labeled, identified, stored, and ultimately linked to the unfortunate patient who coughed it up.

TB strains are labeled alphabetically. Kreiswirth's team began with A. The most common strain that has been found so far in the United States is called W; it was the twenty-third strain identified in the lab. As techniques grew more sophisticated, it became clear that there were different varieties of strain W and other strains. These similar but not identical strains are labeled W1, W2, W3, and so on, and this group of related strains is called the W family.

DNA fingerprinting is an immensely powerful tool that can reveal unsuspected epidemics as well as patterns of disease spread. The technique was developed in 1984 by the British geneticist Alec J. Jeffreys of the University of Leicester and was used to identify people involved in criminal and war crimes cases, based on samples of blood, semen, and other body substances. Later, the technique was used to identify different strains of bacteria.

When Kreiswirth did DNA fingerprinting on the TB bacteria that the New York City Department of Health sent him, he found that the fingerprint exactly matched the W148 strain of TB bacteria, which is the dominant strain in the prison population in Tomsk in Siberia. W148 is almost always resistant to the four-drug standard treatment regimen. Kreiswirth called the city health department and predicted that the patient was Russian and had multi-drug-resistant TB. He was right. The patient was indeed from the former Soviet Union. However, he had only lived in an area thousands of miles away from Tomsk. How could he have the Tomsk prison strain? The only possible answer was that this multi-drug-resistant TB strain was spreading out of the Russian prisons and around the world. It had made its way to Brooklyn, New York; it was just a matter of time before more of the same strain showed up elsewhere.

DNA Fingerprinting Tells Tales

Deadly bacteria enter Barry Kreiswirth's lab daily, arriving nestled inside tightly sealed sturdy brown cardboard boxes about 6 inches on each side. His colleague at the New Jersey Medical School, Dr. Nancy Connell, an associate professor of microbiology, demonstrated the ease with which these dangerous bacteria can be carefully transported. For a program on biowarfare filmed by CNN, the cable news network, using properly approved and appropriate packaging precautions, she carried TB bacteria from her lab in Newark, New Jersey, to Kreiswirth's lab in New York on a regular commuter train. That was before Connell's biosafety level 3 (BSL-3) lab was completed, so that she can now do her own DNA fingerprinting of TB bacteria.

A Russian postdoctoral student in Kreiswirth's lab had brought a well-sealed box of TB bacteria in her hand luggage when she returned from Moscow. A label with Kreiswirth's identification number and a permit from the Centers for Disease Control and Prevention pasted on the outside of the box allowed his lab to receive the deadly bacteria. Such boxes come from all over the world, brought by hand, by delivery service, or by ordinary mail. If something goes wrong, a tracing system will quickly show where the sample came from. The samples in this particular brown box came from the Khomenko institute (the Central TB Research Institute) in Moscow, where TB samples from all over Russia are gathered, tested for susceptibility to anti-tuberculosis drugs, and sent to the Public Health Research Institute for fingerprinting and entry into its database.

Kreiswirth is a very smart, high-energy, fast-talking, informal guy. On the day the box from Moscow arrived, he was wearing his usual office attire: a worn T-shirt promoting Moscow's art and music scene, beat-up gray jeans, and scruffy running shoes. He picked up the box and crossed the hall to enter the BSL-3 lab, where samples of live TB bacteria can be opened.

A BSL-3 lab is designed and built to allow researchers to work safely with dangerous airborne microbes. It must meet many safety regulations. It must be locked at all times, with access controlled by a coded keypad. It must have an anteroom where workers can change into appropriate protective clothing. It must have negative air pressure, so that air flows only into the lab, not out into the rest of the building. The lab must have ultraviolet lights to kill any airborne TB bacteria. It must be painted with special epoxy paint that seals the walls and floors so that no tiny crack remains open. It must have special air filters to catch small and dangerous particles like live TB bacteria.

Kreiswirth punched in the code and opened the steel door from the hall to the anteroom. He then closed the anteroom door as the air flowed gently and silently in from the hall. The door to the lab cannot be opened unless the door to the hall is shut, making the anteroom somewhat like the airlock on a space station.

Putting the box down for a moment, Kreisworth climbed into a white protective coverall sometimes nicknamed a bunny suit. It's made of a tough material similar to that used for those white plastic mailing envelopes you can't rip up. He put surgical booties over his shoes. Over his hands he pulled a double set of latex gloves. Finally, he carefully fitted a protective respirator over his nose and mouth. Although it looks like a simple surgical mask, the respirator forms an airtight seal to keep out deadly bacteria.

At last Kreiswirth carried the cardboard box through the inner door from the anteroom to the BSL-3 lab. Again, the air flowed smoothly past him from the anteroom into the lab as the door closed. Air flowing out of the biosafety lab must pass through high-efficiency particulate air (HEPA) filters, which capture any stray bacteria. As an added safety measure, the air in the lab is forced out through these filters 23 times an hour, a huge number of air changes. An ordinary hospital room's air is changed 6 times per hour; that in a morgue is usually changed 10 times per hour. The lab's air system is checked every 6 months by a team of experts. Every 3 to 5 years the HEPA filters must be replaced, which is done by a decontamination team that comes in wearing protective outfits that look like a cross between a space suit and scuba gear. They gas the bacteria in the filters, then remove the inactivated filters and take them away in special bags.

Kreiswirth's lab has never had a problem in its 9 years of existence, but it stays prepared. If there were to be an accidental spill, the lab would decontaminate itself. Within a few hours, any TB bacteria floating in the air would either be killed by the ultraviolet lights or be sucked into the filters. Ordinarily, the ultraviolet lights stay on all night. Alarms would sound if there were a problem with the negative air pressure. If there were an electrical blackout, the lab would be powered by its own generator. As an additional precaution, inside the biosafety lab, cultures of live TB bacteria are opened only under a biosafety hood, which resembles a large cabinet. The air pressure under the hood is even lower than that in the lab, so that if any TB bacteria are released, they will be sucked up into the HEPA filters in the biosafety hood. Kreiswirth's lab has three of these biosafety cabinets, each a big steel box about 4 feet long and about 7 feet high, with a workspace in front that is partially closed by a clear plastic pane that slides up and down, protecting the worker.

Working under the hood, Kreiswirth finally opened the cardboard box from Moscow. Inside, wrapped in rolls of corrugated cardboard, was a sturdy translucent white plastic container with a screw-on orange top. It looked like a larger, stronger version of the quart ice cream containers in a supermarket freezer. These containers are tough. They can be autoclaved, frozen, or baked, and can be used again and again and again. This one would be going back to Russia, or to some other place that sends TB samples to the lab for analysis.

Inside the plastic container were about 60 hardened glass vials with caps, each about the size of your little toe and housing deadly TB bacteria coughed up by a different patient. The live bacteria were growing on a solid culture medium called a Lowenstein-Jensen slant, after the scientists who developed it. The tubes are slanted to provide a larger surface on which to grow the TB bacteria. The little colonies of TB bacteria looked like breadcrumbs.

Working from one vial at a time, Kreiswirth made a culture of the TB bacteria in each, which he kept in frozen storage in case he should need to check back against the original culture. It is important to work with live bacteria. If he were relying only on dried DNA from Russia, although it is noninfectious, it would be difficult to do an accurate look-back study. If the DNA had been labeled incorrectly in Russia, there would be no way to recheck the original culture of the patient's TB bacteria. So Kreiswirth kept a frozen sample of the TB bacteria. Then he killed the remaining TB bacteria in each sample by heating the sample to 80 degrees Celsius for 30 minutes.

Proceeding with the fingerprinting process, Kreiswirth used chemicals to break open the dead TB cells and isolate the DNA within, which was no longer dangerous. "It's a powder. It looks like dried snot," Kreiswirth said. Since the DNA is not infectious, Kreiswirth and his team are free to work with it in an ordinary lab, without the need for HEPA filters, negative air pressure, and protective clothing. The fingerprinting process usually takes about a week, but it can be done in 3 days if speed is essential. Each sample is kept separate, although several can be processed at one time.

The TB genome was sequenced several years ago. The Sanger Centre in England and The Institute for Genomic Research in the United States sequenced the genome of two different strains of TB. That work makes it possible for scientists to look for mutations in particular parts of the genome.

DNA fingerprinting uses a technique called Southern blotting, named after the scientist who invented it, E. M. Southern. If you think of the circular TB genome as a clock face and the genes as millisecond markings around the clock, then the Southern blot technique is a search for specific millisecond markings, called IS6110 insertions. (IS stands for "insertion sequence.") IS6110 insertions are random bits of DNA that are found in many bacteria. They have the ability to insert themselves into the genome of the cell and make copies of themselves. Nobody knows quite what they do. Different strains of TB bacteria may have anywhere from 0 to 30 IS6110 insertions, and the patterns of IS6110 insertions can tell experts like Kreiswirth how one TB strain differs from another. When Kreiswirth has finished his fingerprinting, the insertions will reveal patterns rather like supermarket bar codes in the different strains of TB bacteria. Just as a bar code reveals that a supermarket item is soap and not baby food, so the IS6110 pattern reveals that one TB bacterial strain is a member of the W family and another is a member of the A family.

The first step in the process is to break up the DNA of the TB from each patient. Each sample is dissolved in a buffer solution until it forms a viscous liquid. Next, a restriction enzyme is added to the liquid. The enzyme cuts the patient's long strand of TB DNA only at certain points. The result is invisible small DNA fragments of different lengths called restriction fragment length polymorphisms (RFLPs).

Next, the fragments are sorted by size, or "run on a gel," as scientists say. Each patient's sliced-up DNA is placed in a separate lane on an electrophoresis gel. This is a plastic plate about the size of a sheet of typing paper, with 10 or 15 lanes, like the lanes for swimmers in a pool. An electric current is applied to the plate and directs the migration of the fragments. The pieces of DNA with the highest molecular weight sluggishly stay near the top of the lane, while the smaller, lighter ones race toward the bottom.

This step separates all the fragments of the entire genome from each patient's TB bacteria. To create the fingerprint, the DNA is transferred, or "blotted" (hence the name Southern blot), onto a membrane. Then a probe of radioactively labeled IS6110 is added. The probe seeks out and attaches to each IS6110 segment in the patient's sample. The places where the radioactively labeled IS6110 probe have attached to IS6110 in the patient's DNA show up as dark bars in each lane on the membrane, literally creating a bar code that can be read and decoded by scientists like Kreiswirth. The placement of the bars from top to bottom is crucial. This striped pattern identifies a particular strain of TB bacteria, which then may be compared to any one of the 12,000 patterns stored in Kreiswirth's database. The comparison, which is made by a powerful computer, shows whether strains are identical twins or kissing cousins or not relatives at all. If there is an identical match (i.e., the two are the same organism), there is a strong likelihood that the infection spread from one individual to the other, or that both were infected by the same source case.

Kreiswirth is particularly interested in the strain W family, sometimes called the Beijing family, because many strains were found in that city. This strain is common throughout East Asia, in China, Taiwan, Singapore, Thailand, Vietnam, Tibet, and also in Russia. Strain W was the predominant strain in the TB epidemic in New York City in the late 1980s and early 1990s. Kreiswirth considers it a "very successful" strain, meaning that it seems to spread easily. It may be more virulent, meaning that it infects people in 24 hours, or it may be more pathogenic, meaning that it is more likely to cause disease; or maybe it is more fit to survive.

Uncovering Epidemics

Fingerprinting DNA can reveal secrets. It can identify strains of tuberculosis that are almost by definition resistant to all first-line drugs, like the strain W148 that Kreiswirth found in the sample from the New York City

Department of Health. In recent years, fingerprinting has enabled us to identify epidemics that would otherwise have gone unrecognized. For instance,
one-third to one-half of TB cases in some U.S. cities occur in clusters, groups
of patients whose TB bacteria have the same DNA pattern. That suggests
recent infection with TB, acquired from a single source rather than reactivation of old, latent infections that were probably acquired years ago, somewhere else. If the cases were due to reactivation, the DNA patterns would
most likely be quite different.

DNA fingerprinting told us an interesting story that no one would have
suspected right in Newark, at the New Jersey Medical School National TB
Center.[1] We knew that coughing is not the only way in which TB can be
spread, although it is the most common. Any aerosol can do the trick—like
singing, for instance. Singing sends fewer droplets containing TB bacteria into
the air, but the droplets may be smaller and hang in the air longer.

There is a local church in Newark, New Jersey, that has well-known
gospel choirs; they even sang for President Bill Clinton during his 1996
reelection campaign. Its members meet frequently to rehearse, and many of
them are also friends who share rides to and from choir practice.

In June 1995, the New Jersey state health department investigated two
cases of active TB in the same local law firm. They did conventional contact tracing, seeking out the people with whom each patient spent most of
his or her time and skin-testing them for TB. However, the two patients at
the law firm were not in contact with each other at the workplace, nor did
they live in the same community. Later we found a third case of active TB
from a different town, in a patient with no connection with the law firm.
This patient was initially diagnosed elsewhere and then referred to us.

Each of the three active cases had been reported to the state TB registry from a different township. After extensive interviews and investigation,
state TB officials were unable to make a connection among the cases. The
only thing the three patients had in common was that they sang in one of
the gospel choirs at that church in Newark. The state asked for our help.
We got an old list of more than 500 choir members and matched it to the
current state TB registry (an official list of TB cases). We found two more
active cases, including the probable source case, a homeless man who lived
in a shelter. He was the church custodian and also sang in the choir.

Four of the five people with active TB were tenors (including two
women) and sang in the 11 A.M. choir. The tenor section was in an area where
air flowed up from vents in the floor and, we think, spread the TB bacteria
backward. This would explain why none of the sopranos, who sat directly
in front of the tenors but on the other side of the floor vents, had caught

TB. Several other choir members did have positive tuberculin skin tests, indicating infection, but they did not have active TB, so we could not test them to find out if they had been infected recently or were infected many years ago. Tenors were twice as likely as other choir members to have positive skin tests. Since we could never know *when* they had been infected, we followed our standard practice of offering treatment to everyone with a positive skin test.

Of the five choir members with active tuberculosis, we were able to have DNA fingerprinting done on TB strains for four; the fifth had TB outside the lungs, and so we could not easily get a sample of the bacteria. All of the choir members who had active TB had the same strain of TB except one, known as Case Number Three, a woman who sang alto in the 11 A.M. choir. She had TB all right, but DNA fingerprinting showed that she did not have the same strain of TB as the other members of the choir. Obviously she had contracted her TB from another source. Only DNA fingerprinting could have told us this. Without it, we would just have thought she was part of the church choir outbreak.

Another surprise was Case Number Four, who had the same strain of TB as the members of the 11 A.M. choir but sang only in the 8 A.M. choir. How did she become infected? The most likely answer was that she occasionally commuted with one of the choir members with who was a member of the 11 A.M. choir.

In a group of middle-aged individuals (the patients were aged 38 to 62), it would be natural to assume that active TB was a reactivation of an old, latent infection. However, DNA fingerprinting of this outbreak told us that in these cases the same strain of TB had likely been recently transmitted from one individual to the others. If the patients had reactivation of old latent infections, the strains would have been different. Furthermore, with the exception of the homeless man who served as church custodian, this TB outbreak was not among poor and socially deprived individuals, but among middle-class, employed people whose recreational interest was singing in a nationally known church choir. These cases could easily have been missed by traditional contact tracing, which is designed to look for cases among those who spend a lot of time with a patient, such as the family. Fingerprinting the choir mini-epidemic showed us that social networks could be quite important in transmitting TB.

Linking cases and finding unsuspected outbreaks would be much easier if we did DNA fingerprinting of every case of pulmonary TB, as is done in the Netherlands. There, the fingerprint analysis is available to public health

workers, who trace contacts of patients with active tuberculosis and iden-
tify the sometimes unsuspected links in TB transmission, according to Dr.
Kitty Lambregts, the former coordinator of program support for the Royal
Netherlands TB Association (known as KNCV, for its initials in Dutch).

A "Down Home" Problem

Just about the last place in the United States where you'd expect to find an
outbreak of an astonishingly virulent form of tuberculosis would be in the
rural communities on the border between Kentucky and Tennessee. But
there were many unusual aspects to the outbreak that occurred in 1995 in
two counties there, with a combined population of about 14,000. Each
county had had fewer than one case of TB per year before the outbreak.[2]
From a scientist's point of view, the Tennessee-Kentucky outbreak was a good
case to study because the infection routes were so clear and because there
had previously been so little TB in the area.[3] This outbreak stood out like a
sore thumb, and DNA fingerprinting revealed its secrets.

The investigation presented many surprises. We knew that it was possible to get TB on an 8-hour airline flight, but we felt pretty secure that infection following brief contact was very unusual. That's why TB experts usually
told reporters, "Yes, you can get it on the subway, but the chances are higher
that the subway will crash." This rural outbreak showed that TB could be
transmitted at a holiday dinner with family, if one of the group had active
TB. It was a frightening thought. Did it mean that people could get TB in
fleeting everyday situations, like on the bus or the subway?

The index case—let's call him Charlie—was a young man, which was
unusual in itself. In a small, stable rural community like this, tuberculosis is
likely to occur mainly in the elderly, where it is usually the reactivation of
an old latent infection. The people in this community were all born in the
United States, so their tuberculin skin test results could not be confused by
any prior BCG vaccination, as this is virtually never done in the United
States.

In the autumn of 1994, about a month before Charlie started work at
a nearby garment factory, he saw a doctor because he had chest pains and
a cough. The doctor diagnosed pneumonia and prescribed antibiotics, which
seemed to help for a while. Charlie went to work at the local garment factory. It was a huge barnlike room with a high ceiling. It had excellent air circulation, but not a lot of incoming fresh air—an ideal situation for spreading
TB bacteria. Workers sat at workstations about 5 or 6 feet apart, sewing

garments. About a month after he started work, Charlie went back to see the doctor because he still had a cough; the doctor gave him another antibiotic. In the early winter of 1995, he went back to the doctor again. This time he was prescribed cough medicine.

In April 1995, 6 or 7 months after Charlie first went to his doctor with chest symptoms, his young niece was given a tuberculin skin test for tuberculosis as part of a regular school checkup, and the test was positive. Alarm bells went off. Public health workers from the Centers for Disease Control and the Tennessee and Kentucky health departments moved in. The whole family was screened. Charlie was found to have active tuberculosis, and the disease, which had gone undiagnosed for so many months, had created large cavities full of TB bacteria in his lungs, a highly infectious state.

The public health workers went looking for other people whom Charlie might have infected, and for the person who might have infected Charlie. They searched state TB registries for people from the area who had TB. They searched pharmacy records to find people who were taking TB medications. In addition to Charlie's family, they gave tuberculin skin tests to his coworkers in the garment factory and his social contacts, whether they were close or casual.

The public health workers were surprised by the size of the skin reactions of people who had been exposed to Charlie's TB. A positive skin test reaction is usually about the size of a dime, but these positive skin test reactions were twice as big. Some even showed up as blisters, which is uncommon. Puzzled, the public health workers checked the lot of the TB test substance (purified protein derivative) to see if there was something unusual about it. There wasn't. It seemed that Charlie's TB was so virulent that it caused extreme reactions.

Charlie's TB was also unusually good at infecting people. Every single one of Charlie's family and close friends had a positive skin test. So did 71 percent of his coworkers in the garment factory. And, amazingly, so were 46 percent of his casual contacts, and some of these were very casual. The only contact some people had had with Charlie was socializing in the evening outside the local gas station. TB transmission in the open air is very rare.

Five people developed active TB; among them were two of Charlie's relatives, who could have been infected only during the 3 hours they spent with him at Christmas or Easter dinner. They had had absolutely no other contact with him and lived miles away.

Later, 10 more cases of active TB turned up in the county where Charlie lived. Among them were a mother and her 2-year-old child who had merely been waiting in the same private doctor's office with one of the other cases. The doctor's office staff was skin-tested. Half of them were skin-test-positive, indicating TB infection, when they had been negative before. Again, it was astonishing that such brief exposure led to transmission of TB.

DNA fingerprinting of everyone with active TB showed that they had exactly the same strain Charlie had. They hadn't caught it from someone else or experienced a reactivation of an old latent infection. Clearly, Charlie's strain of TB was extraordinarily infectious. When scientists infected mice with the strain, it grew hundreds of times more rapidly than other virulent strains of TB. The good news was that Charlie's TB strain was sensitive to the four first-line drugs used in standard TB treatment.

Many questions remain: Where did Charlie get his TB? How much more of this virulent TB was floating around Kentucky and Tennessee in people who had not been linked to Charlie, his family, his coworkers, or his buddies despite the careful investigation? The CDC widened its search to surrounding counties and did DNA fingerprinting on the 25 cases of TB that had been reported from there. No luck. None of the 25 cases had the same DNA fingerprint as Charlie's TB. According to Dr. Ida Onorato, who was in charge of the investigation of this outbreak and was, until recently, the head of TB surveillance at CDC, to this day nobody knows where Charlie got his TB. Thanks to DNA fingerprinting, however, CDC was able to distinguish this strain of TB from random cases of reactivated TB.

A Step toward Treatment That Works

DNA fingerprinting identifies related strains of TB bacteria, and scientists know from experience that certain strains are almost always multi-drug-resistant, like the strain Kreiswirth identified from the Russian immigrant in Brooklyn. However, when multi-drug resistance is common, as it is in Russia, only drug-sensitivity testing will give the doctor a definitive answer on what antibiotics will cure the patient's disease and what antibiotics are useless. If the doctor doesn't have this crucial information, the patient is likely to get the wrong treatment, which almost invariably encourages the development of resistance to more drugs: The patient who started out with TB that was resistant to one or two drugs may end up with TB that is resistant to three or four drugs and can transmit that even more drug-resistant TB.

Drug-susceptibility testing takes anywhere from three weeks (if the scientist is in a hurry and has funds for a fast-track approach) to 3 months or more. In Russia so far, drug-susceptibility testing is seldom available, even though it is obviously essential to controlling that nation's TB epidemic.

When I give lectures, I sometimes show a slide of the clinical course of a typical multi-drug-resistant TB patient. It shows the complicated cycles of drug-susceptibility studies and the changes in drug regimens that were prescribed until, at last, the physicians taking care of this patient finally discovered what drugs would cure him. Unfortunately, he had died a month before.

9

Epidemic in New York

On February 10, 1999, an icy cold but brilliantly clear and sunny day, General Vladimir Yalunin, the new head of the Russian prison system, made a visit to Rikers Island, the pretrial detention center and jail that is the heart of New York City's prison system. He was accompanied by members of his medical and administrative staff and by people from George Soros's Open Society Institute and the Public Health Research Institute, which, with funds from the Open Society Institute, had paid for his trip. His visit was chronicled by David Remnick, editor of *The New Yorker*, who had previously reported from Moscow and knew the Russian situation.[1]

General Yalunin wanted to learn how New York had conquered its epidemic of multi-drug-resistant tuberculosis in the late 1980s and early 1990s. The city's epidemic had been centered in its jails, such as those on Rikers Island, and had spread to hospitals, just like the much smaller outbreak in the upstate New York prison which killed the Syracuse prison guard. In 1992, the worst year of the epidemic, New York City had 3,811 cases of TB in a population of 7 1/2 million; 441 of the patients had multi-drug-resistant TB.[2] A few hundred people died, mostly those who were also infected with HIV/AIDS.

Back in Russia, General Yalunin faced an infinitely worse situation. In order to gain admittance to the Council of Europe, Russia had agreed to improve conditions for its prisoners, so the administration of the entire prison system had been transferred from the Ministry of the Interior to the Ministry of Justice, and Yalunin had been put in charge of GUIN, the prison system. Therefore, Yalunin was now responsible for more than a million prisoners in Russia's pretrial detention centers, prisons, and TB colonies—the system Russians still call the Gulag. Yalunin knew that if he could make the prison system work against TB, as the New Yorkers did, he would go a long way toward protecting the Russian population as well as people around the world.

Of Yalunin's 1 million prisoners, about 100,000 had active, infectious tuberculosis. Even more alarming, at least 20,000 to 30,000 of them had multi-drug-resistant tuberculosis. And the prisons had not yet felt even a hint of the coming Russian AIDS epidemic. With only 3811 cases in its worst year, New York City's epidemic had been tiny by comparison, but Yalunin wanted to see how the city had successfully controlled its epidemic and how it was currently handling TB in the prisons and jails.

As in Russia, the TB epidemic in New York had been centered in the prison system. When TB-infected prisoners, some of whom also were infected with HIV, which made them 800 times more susceptible to active TB, were hospitalized, the disease spread to vulnerable hospital workers, some of whom also were infected with HIV. Some of the hospital workers may have known of their HIV infection, but many probably did not. Some suffered devastating, fulminating cases of active TB. Some patients died within a few weeks. Outbreaks of multi-drug-resistant TB occurred in seven New York City hospitals; the mortality rate among these patients was over 80 percent.[3] All of these frightening elements—TB, multi-drug-resistant TB, quickly rising HIV rates—were right there on Yalunin's doorstep in Russia.

On Rikers Island

It's not easy to get to Rikers Island even if you have been arrested. The only entrance is over a steeply humped two-lane bridge from Queens, one of the five boroughs of New York City, and through a rigorous check at an official booth. Named for an early Dutch settler, Abraham Riker, the island holds 10 of New York City's 16 jails.

Anybody who has flown into or out of La Guardia Airport in New York has probably flown over Rikers Island without noticing it. It's a small island, and on the day of Yalunin's visit, the waters of the East River were sparkling in the winter sun. From a distance, the widely spaced prison units looked like garden apartments. Most were four stories tall and built of beige brick; a few were eight stories. But, unlike garden apartments, all the units had bars over every window. The buildings were separated by fences, ribbons of razor wire, and well-tended grass on which Canada geese rested. Inside, the buildings were overheated and rigorously clean, and they had the same stale cafeteria food smells as the halls of your local high school. But they did not smell of unwashed bodies and stale urine, like Russian prisons.

Yalunin was officially greeted by Bernard B. Kerik, the New York City commissioner of corrections. A former police officer, Kerik had succeeded in reducing violence in the jail, which had suffered from frequent riots and attacks by inmates on other prisoners and guards. He took charge after the TB epidemic had been contained, but he was proud of Rikers Island's rigorous control of TB among prisoners. (He later became New York City's police commissioner.) The meeting took place in Kerik's headquarters, a small two-story house probably built in the 1940s that had been converted into offices. Outside, parked near the bright blue waters, were riot-control vehicles, including a tank. Yalunin, a stocky man in his late 40s, climbed into the tank for a photo opportunity.

Rikers Island is the largest jail in the United States.[4] It holds about 17,000 inmates who are awaiting trial or serving short sentences. Most are confined for about 6 or 7 weeks. Thus, Rikers Island is akin to the SIZOs of Russia, the pretrial detention centers that hold people who have been arrested and whose cases are being investigated. In the New York City TB epidemic, the city improved TB screening of inmates at Rikers Island and built a unique, safe, and very expensive Communicable Disease Unit there, in which prisoners with TB or other infectious diseases could be isolated and treated. Now, inmates are screened for TB with skin tests or chest X-rays when they first enter the facility. If there is any suspicion of TB, they are isolated in these special units, as are inmates who have known active TB or other infectious diseases, are suspected of having TB, or have not complied with treatment for TB. Inmates with TB receive directly observed therapy to cure their disease.

The isolation units are called "sprung units" because they are sprung from a central supporting structure, rather like an umbrella sitting on the ground. It is a relatively inexpensive and quick way to build, but the final cost is high because of the precautions needed to prevent the spread of infectious diseases. The units are connected in clusters. Inside the Communicable Disease Unit are 140 isolation units. Each isolation unit costs about $250,000 and holds one prisoner.

Anyone entering a patient's locked isolation unit, such as the nurse who provides directly observed therapy, must first go into a glass-walled anteroom. Only when the entry door from the hallway has closed can the person open the door from the anteroom to the cell itself. Each cell is under negative pressure, so that air can flow only from the corridor into the anteroom, through the patient's cell, and then out through high-efficiency particulate air (HEPA) filters to the outside, where sunlight will kill any remaining bugs. The filters themselves are removed and sanitized at frequent intervals. The system, which is very similar to Barry Kreiswirth's system at PHRI for laboratory researchers, is designed to protect health-care workers. Each cell has 10 air changes per hour, and the negative pressure is monitored

24 hours a day. Each prisoner's cell is small, clean, and efficient, about 120 square feet (10 feet by 12 feet). Almost everything but the mattress is stainless steel, which can be scrubbed and sterilized easily. There's a single bed, a washbasin, a shower, a toilet, a table or bookshelf, and a TV suspended from the wall.

Staff workers told Yalunin and his team that they felt safer here in the Communicable Disease Unit, where they know what the risks and the protections are, than in places where prisoners have not yet been tested for TB. All new correction officers [guards] are skin-tested for TB to see if they have had a previous TB infection. Those who work in areas where they may be exposed to TB, like the people in the Communicable Disease Units, get skin-tested every 6 months to detect a change from their previous test, which could only be caused by a new infection. Demonstrating the effectiveness of these units, since they have been in use, no staff member had "converted" —that is, developed a positive skin test after previous negative ones—by the time of Yalunin's visit.

Yalunin looked around him with appreciation and amazement. Back home, he had less than a dollar a day to take care of each Russian prison inmate, and his budget was being cut. He had prisoners crammed into cells so crowded that they had to sleep in shifts. He had no safeguards like negative air pressure for prisoners or for his guards and medical staff, not even simple protective masks or even simple, basic procedures like skin testing. He didn't have even a fraction of the money it would take to build such a facility to hold and treat TB patients. He needed funds for TB drugs, for beds for prisoners with TB, for laboratories. He had a lot to think about when he returned to Russia.

Timebomb in Times Square

In the 1980s, the timebomb of multi-drug-resistant tuberculosis exploded in New York City. By 1992, although New York had only 3 percent of the U.S. population of 270 million, its 3811 TB cases were 14 percent of U.S. TB cases and 61 percent of the multi-drug-resistant cases in the entire country. It was an epidemic, but an exceedingly small one compared to what is happening in Russia today. When public health authorities finally recognized the problem in New York, they not only threw money at it but they were fortunate enough to enlist young, smart, energetic, and knowledgeable professionals. The epidemic shook public health experts and cost the city and the nation's taxpayers $1 billion in excess health expenditures. Most of all, it was an expensive lesson in what happens when routine but *essential* public health vigilance is neglected.

Journalists, scientists, and doctors are wrong when they refer to the New York City tuberculosis epidemic as the epidemic of the late 1980s and the early 1990s. The New York City epidemic really began in 1972. In that year, TB experts were celebrating the fact that TB cases had been going down as a result of good public health measures and the new, powerful drug treatment regimens. Essentially, the effort against TB had been so successful that Congress decided that we didn't need it any longer. In 1972, despite protests from people who were deeply committed to finally eradicating TB, Congress voted to convert funds that had been strictly designated for TB control and elimination into so-called block grants that states could use for any purpose they wanted. Most states chose to cut or eliminate their funding for TB control and to use the money for more politically appealing priorities. Thanks to the switch to block grants, TB stopped getting much attention in New York City. Through this increasing neglect, New York City was building a timebomb through the 1970s and 1980s.

In 1968, about $40 million was spent on TB treatment and control in New York City; by 1978, funding had dropped to between $23 million and $25 million. By 1979, New York City had lost almost all its federal funding; New York State, which had provided half the money for the city's work against TB, cut off all funds. By 1978, the city was spending much less than $2 million on TB control and treatment.[5] Also during this period, New York suffered its most serious financial crisis, when the city failed in its appeal for help to President Gerald Ford in Washington. The *Daily News* ran its famous headline: "Ford to City: Drop Dead."

The city health department's Bureau of Tuberculosis Control was down to its lowest staff level ever. There were only about 10 outreach workers to respond to the 7000 or 8000 suspected tuberculosis cases reported every year. These workers were unable to make sure that people with active TB were taking their medicines and not infecting family, friends, and colleagues. Instead, they were spending their time screening people for TB infection with skin tests, just as the Russians, in a similar way, try to X-ray the entire population at frequent intervals to find TB. The 24 health department chest clinics had been cut to 8, and all the combined public health and chest clinics in city and voluntary hospitals had been closed.[6] Before the cutoff of funds, the city had had 1000 beds for TB patients, mostly in municipal hospitals that treat the poor and desperate, who are more likely to need hospital care. Now, in crisis time, the city had about 100 TB beds, and almost none of them were in isolation units that would protect hospital staff from infection.

Meanwhile, during the 1980s the city was suffering from an economic recession, a growing epidemic of HIV/AIDS, and a surge of immigrants, legal and illegal, from countries that had high tuberculosis rates. Homelessness was common. Men slept in cardboard boxes in the doorways of jewelry stores and boutiques on Madison Avenue, the city's most stylish and expensive shopping street. They slept on grates outside the Museum of Modern Art and near Grand Central Station, where warm air came up from subterranean sources, just as some Russian homeless people slept near the huge heating pipes in Tomsk. Some went to the city's shelters for the homeless. The shelters were huge, overcrowded, dangerous institutions that accommodated hundreds of people and were very effective at spreading TB.

Also during the 1980s, the HIV/AIDS virus had become widespread in the city's gay community and among intravenous drug users, their sex partners, and their children, although many did not know they were infected. Over 40 percent of patients with TB in the city also had AIDS or HIV infection. People who are infected with HIV/AIDS are 800 times more likely to develop active TB from a recent or past latent TB infection than other people. In addition, immigrants, many of them illegal, were arriving from countries where tuberculosis was common, such as Mexico, the Philippines, the former Soviet Union, Vietnam, Haiti, El Salvador, India, the Dominican Republic, and mainland China.

For a while the New York City TB rate held steady. Then, beginning around 1979, it began to surge upward. By 1992, it had almost tripled. The system wasn't working anymore. TB patients who had been so ill that they needed hospital care never completed their treatment. They walked out of the hospital feeling better and clutching a prescription—and disappeared. Dr. Jay Dobkin and Dr. Karen Brudney of Harlem Hospital and Columbia-Presbyterian Medical Center found that *89 percent* of the TB patients who had been discharged from Harlem Hospital never completed their required treatment. Of course, that didn't mean that they were cured. After brief treatment, they probably felt better and stopped taking their pills. Then they probably got sick again, spread TB to their families, friends, and colleagues —particularly if they lived in one of the huge, crowded shelters—and eventually came back to a hospital with TB that was now resistant to the usual antibiotics.

Almost no one noticed the development of increased multi-drug-resistant TB, except Dobkin and Brudney and my old colleague Dr. Charles Felton, the TB expert at Harlem Hospital. With the decline in funds for TB investigation and treatment, plus the social and economic problems, Felton saw that the TB rates in central Harlem had reached 240 cases per 100,000 people, which was higher than in many Third World countries. But Felton's protests fell on deaf ears.

The Timebomb Explodes

The job of health commissioner of New York City has been called the most important public health job in the country. The position has been filled by legendary figures in public health, such as Hermann Biggs. At the turn of the twentieth century, Biggs began New York's seminal effort against tuberculosis, then the leading cause of death in an overcrowded, heavily immigrant city.

The new New York City health commissioner in 1991 was Dr. Margaret Hamburg, a brilliantly effective but unassuming young woman whom everyone just called Peggy. She recruited a team of bright young doctors and hundreds of unsung workers in the trenches. She was the youngest health commissioner ever, and only the third woman to hold the job. Although she was only in her early thirities, Hamburg already had major credentials. She had graduated from Harvard College and Harvard Medical School and was board-certified in internal medicine. She had worked at the federal Department of Health and Human Services and the National Institute of Allergy and Infectious Diseases of the National Institutes of Health. She had interests in drug addiction, primary care, women's health, and the international spread of disease. It was a blessing that she had an easy but calm and thoughtful manner and was able to present hardened politicians with careful plans on what to do about the TB epidemic.

When Hamburg took charge in 1991 and looked at the situation, she unearthed something far worse than an epidemic of plain old tuberculosis: an epidemic of multi-drug-resistant tuberculosis. She had a snapshot study of TB cases during April 1991 done by Dr. Tom Frieden, who was on loan from the Centers for Disease Control and Pevention. The results took Hamburg and her colleagues by surprise.

Frieden's study showed that one-third of New York's TB patients had a strain that was resistant to one or more drugs. Among patients who had previously been treated for TB, 44 percent now had tuberculosis that was resistant to one or more drugs. That meant that their previous treatment had been inadequate or incomplete, fostering resistance. Worse yet, of patients who had never been treated for TB, 23 percent had TB that was resistant to at least one drug, up from 10 percent only a few years before. These patients didn't have drug-resistant TB because of inadequate treatment. They had drug-resistant TB because they had caught it from somebody with drug-resistant TB. In other words, drug-resistant TB was spreading throughout the city.[7]

Hamburg and her colleagues put together a plan and persuaded the mayor, David Dinkins, to make the campaign against tuberculosis a priority. They convinced him and state and federal health authorities that greatly increased funds were needed to deal with New York City's epidemic, and they worked tirelessly with Dinkins and other officials to make sure that money to combat TB was included in each city agency's budget. Hamburg recalled, "I could just have thrown my hands up and said to the mayor, 'We have a problem . . . poverty, HIV, we don't have a handle on either one,' and he might have moved on. He would have thought, 'Yes, it's terrible,' but we'd have been left behind. Having something concrete to offer was essential. We had the ability to present a clearly defined program that could make a difference relatively quickly. The great thing we did in New York was to define a set of goals and objectives."

Federal funding for TB control in New York City shot up from about $5 million a year to about $35 million. As evidence that the city recognized the problem and was committed to curing it, the city put $100 million of its own funds into the fight in 1992.[8]

In an extraordinary piece of public health work (which I consider one of the great public health victories of the twentieth century), Hamburg and her colleagues managed to turn the epidemic around, assisted in large part by the political will sought by Hamburg and readily provided by the enlightened mayor and his senior aides. In recognition of her work, Mayor Dinkins gave Dr. Hamburg a desk plaque that reads "Czarina." She had it still, on her desk in her office overlooking Capitol Hill and the Mall, when she was assistant secretary of health for planning and evaluation at the Department of Health and Human Services during the Clinton administration, where her responsibilities included the national security threat posed by infectious diseases such as TB that fly across borders.

Ending the Epidemic in New York

On Hamburg's team were two young physicians on loan from the Centers for Disease Control and Prevention, Drs. Thomas Frieden and Paula Fujiwara. They were among the 20 people that the CDC recruited to help get multidrug-resistant TB under control in New York. Fujiwara, an internal medicine expert from California, arrived in March 1992, the worst year of the epidemic. "It was a very, very dysfunctional system," she recalled. "I was appalled at how poorly run it had been. No one respected us at first. Tom Frieden [who was head of the Bureau of TB Control] and I were reaching out. We gave two, three talks a week to anyone who would listen." They spoke to medical and academic communities, policymakers, hospital discharge planners, and the public. They wrote and distributed leaflets, and they emphasized that directly observed therapy increased patients' chances of being cured. In the medical community, they focused on academics who had previously ignored TB but who had cachet in New York's many famous medical centers. They reasoned that if they could convince respected, forward-thinking academics, these opinion leaders would pass the message on.

Hamburg realized that directly observed therapy (DOT) was the gold standard of care for TB patients and the way to get the epidemic under control. Treating and curing patients with ordinary TB would prevent them from developing multi-drug-resistant TB. Directly observed therapy had actually been used in New York in a very limited way since 1979, for fewer than 100 people, usually homeless individuals and men who lived on the Bowery, New York's Skid Row. For some of these people, outreach workers brought their medicine to them—to cheap hotels or neighborhood bars; other patients came to clinics. But patients had to have a stable address and agree to accept directly observed therapy, and there weren't any bonuses for doing so. If they disappeared from treatment, the staff tried to trace them but often could not find them. When the staff cuts occurred in the years leading up to the epidemic, the tracing effort became even less successful and more frustrating. Fewer than half of all patients completed treatment. The rest were out there, still sick, still infecting their families, friends, and casual contacts.

Directly observed therapy had first been suggested by Dr. John Sbarbaro of the National Jewish Center for Immunology and Respiratory Medicine in Denver in 1973, and my colleague Dr. Reynard McDonald documented its effectiveness in 1982.

A Contract to Care

Under Hamburg's direction, the health department began promoting directly observed therapy as a supportive service to help patients complete their treatment, not as an intrusion or a punishment for being unreliable. The treatment was provided at clinics, which were kept open nights and weekends, or was delivered to the patient at home, at work, or at a convenient place—a bar, a subway station, a ferry terminal, a neighborhood corner, or a crack den.

In each case, the patient, the chest clinic manager, and the physician signed a remarkable contract. The patient agreed to come to all scheduled appointments or to notify the clinic when this wasn't possible, to keep the clinic informed if he or she moved, and to tell the doctor or clinic manager if there were problems with care. In return, the clinic manager agreed that the patient would be in and out of the clinic in 15 minutes, or 90 minutes if he or she had to see a doctor. All medications would be free, and the patient would be reimbursed for transportation to and from the clinic. In addition, the clinic manager agreed to answer any of the patient's questions and to try to provide referrals for social services. The physician in charge agreed to provide the patient with the most advanced and effective therapy and to answer any questions from the patient or the clinic manager.

Patients got incentives to complete treatment: one can of a liquid food supplement each day, a $5 food coupon each week they completed treatment, and the transportation money. Patients who had to receive treatment daily at a clinic got even more incentives: transportation coupons,[9] food coupons, breakfast or lunch, and a graduated package of incentives, up to $60 per month.

The health department made a point of hiring workers who were knowledgeable about and comfortable with the patients they were treating. They looked for people who were bilingual in English and Spanish, Chinese, Haitian Creole, and the languages of the Indian subcontinent, the many tongues spoken in the immigrant community of New York. The workers had to be college graduates, but the starting pay was only about $25,000 a year, which was a very small amount in a very expensive city. Nevertheless, the department found extremely dedicated people who went far, far out of their way to make sure their patients got treated and got better. When a patient died, as some invariably did, the department offered grief counseling to the staff. The doctors themselves were on the front line: Frieden, who directed the program, made a point of seeing TB patients himself in neighborhood clinics. Through periodic reviews of patient records, the progress of *each* patient in the entire city was presented to Frieden and to his successor in the job, Fujiwara.

Meanwhile, TB screening was implemented in city jails and the Communicable Disease Unit that Yalunin visited was built at Rikers Island. Infection control was improved at local hospitals, which began retrofitting rooms with protective negative pressure. The large, dangerous homeless shelters were downsized.

Typhoid Marys

A critical civil rights issue arose: What should the health department do about patients who refused to be treated or who just quit treatment and disappeared? At the turn of the century, Typhoid Mary had spread illness and death to people for whom she worked as a cook. When she refused to stop working, she was imprisoned. That was then. This was a new era, sensitive to civil rights.

Patients with active TB who evaded treatment were even more dangerous than Typhoid Mary. They could spread the disease to anyone who shared their air. Should they be forced into treatment or imprisoned? Some people held that no one should be treated if he or she didn't want to be. Others said that the public should be protected from an airborne disease. TB, they said, was not like AIDS, where you could decide whether or not to engage in risky activity.

In the end, after much advice and discussion, in April 1993 the New York City health code was revised to offer a sensitive solution. The health commissioner could order patients with suspected or proven tuberculosis to be examined and to be treated. If they didn't complete treatment, they could be required to receive directly observed therapy on an outpatient basis. If they had active, infectious TB, they could be detained in a hospital. And, even if they were no longer infectious, they could be detained until they completed the full course of treatment, to prevent the development of multi-drug-resistant TB. Hearings and free legal services were provided to patients. The city opened a 25-bed detention ward for noncompliant TB patients at Goldwater Memorial Hospital on an island in the East River. Although no one can prove it, health officials think the mere threat of detention encouraged patients to comply with less restrictive treatments. In any case, no more than 47 patients were ever detained at any one time in the whole city.

The program in both the city and the jails worked spectacularly, and, I am convinced, saved the city, surrounding states, and the nation from an infectious disease calamity. However, to this day prison or jail inmates who refuse to be tested or treated for TB are represented, at public expense, by private attorneys from high-powered, prestigious law firms, who argue that their civil rights are being infringed. In stark contrast, the public health interest is invariably represented by a principled assistant district attorney or assistant attorney general who may have graduated from law school only recently. Lamentably, the courts don't always find for public health, which may, soon, once again, actually lead to spreading tuberculosis in these facilities.

Deadly Strain W

Meanwhile, the city health department, the Centers for Disease Control, and the Public Health Research Institute were tracing the different strains of tuberculosis that were infecting patients. Finding similar strains might mean that the patients had been exposed to some common source many years ago. Or, far more likely, it might mean that patients had been infected recently.

Barry Kreiswirth and his colleagues from the CDC and several hospitals in New York looked at a particularly vicious strain of multi-drug-resistant tuberculosis. They investigated every case between January 1, 1990, and August 1, 1993, that was resistant to isoniazid, rifampin, ethambutol, and streptomycin. They did drug-susceptibility testing and DNA fingerprinting. There were 357 patients in their study, and 267 of them had identical or close-to-identical DNA fingerprints: strain W.

Almost all of the strain W patients were young Hispanic men, average age about 38, and almost all of them had HIV infection. They came from different areas in the city, and they were treated at 41 different hospitals. Among them were 20 health-care workers, most of whom worked at hospitals where there had been outbreaks of TB within the hospital. Almost all of the patients got infected in a hospital where they were being treated for HIV, in wards where they could spread TB to other patients with HIV infection. Almost all of them died, most without ever leaving the hospital. Often, it was only long after a patient died that doctors learned that he had had TB that was resistant to all the drugs they had been treating him with. This small group of patients with strain W represented one-quarter of all patients with multi-drug-resistant TB in the United States at the time. Kreiswirth and his colleagues have identified strain W as a common strain in Russian prisons and in East Asia. How it got to New York City, nobody knows.

Strain W was not only busy killing patients in hospitals, it was also a hazard to health-care workers and to the doctors battling tuberculosis around the city. Despite precautions, both Frieden and Kreiswirth became skin-test positive for what may be strain W. They were infected but not ill. Both took preventive medication. Both are well—so far.

Converting

"Converting your skin test," as Kreiswirth and Frieden did, is a frightening punch in the stomach. It is a reminder that catching a possibly fatal disease is one of the risks you take for being a doctor or nurse, or just for working in a hospital. At around the same time as Kreiswirth and Frieden converted, so did one of my medical students, Beth Malasky, who can tell what it's like to live with this problem. Beth came to me and told me that her skin test had converted from negative to positive. She knew all about TB, and not just as a medical student. Her sister Charlotte was a pulmonary physician, and so was Charlotte's husband, Paul. They told her, "Don't sweat it. It can be treated."

The problem was that we didn't know what kind of TB Beth had, and so we didn't know how to keep her from getting sick from it. Beth suspected that she had been infected with multi-drug-resistant TB. She thought that the most likely source of her infection was a little Haitian girl, Merlande, who had been in isolation in the pediatric unit at University Hospital in Newark for months with suspected multi-drug-resistant TB. Beth had spent a lot of time playing with Merlande, who was lonely and sick. The child was infected with HIV, and she had caught tuberculosis from her father—a deadly combination. Because of her TB, Merlande had to stay in an isolation room or wear a mask so that she would not spread TB to other patients or to the hospital staff. Visitors like Beth were required to wear a mask to prevent them from getting infected.

Merlande was lonely, and she didn't want to wear her mask, which was hot and stuffy and made breathing difficult. Beth felt sorry for the little girl. She was sick and in pain, and she was isolated; there was nobody to look after her, cuddle her, or play with her. Every chance she got, Beth went to the little girl's room and played with her. Merlande brightened up when Beth came into her room. "She was so sick she could barely stand, but when I came into the room, she'd be standing up in the crib looking through the bars like it was a cage," Beth said. Beth smiled at her and tickled her and brought her coloring books and simple toys. Merlande responded to Beth's attention as any child would: She loved it. She brightened up when Beth came into her room. She smiled and played and hugged Beth and she tried to pull off Beth's mask. Perhaps Beth should have been more careful, but pediatric experts told her she was very unlikely to get TB from a child. "They just don't cough hard enough to send TB bacteria out into the air," she was authoritatively told.

Now Beth's skin test had converted to positive, indicating a latent TB infection. What treatment should she get to prevent her from getting active tuberculosis? It was possible that, despite her contact with Merlande, she might have become infected with ordinary TB from some other patient, perhaps in the emergency room or when she had worked for short periods at other hospitals in New Jersey and at a Native American reservation in the Southwest. Still, Beth was convinced that she had been infected with multi-drug-resistant TB and that she had caught it from Merlande. Because Beth did not have active TB, there was no way we could retrieve the bacteria from her body and do DNA fingerprinting or drug-sensitivity testing on them Because of a laboratory error, Merlande's drug susceptibility tests didn't grow, so they were unable provide this information. Beth knew that if she were to develop active multi-drug-resistant TB, she would have only a 50–50 chance of surviving for 5 years. Given a choice, she would be better off with breast cancer, where there's about a 90 percent chance of surviving for 5 years. Beth didn't get to choose her disease.

What preventive drugs should she take? Even I wasn't sure. I had one of my trainees call 32 expert colleagues across the country. This method is called a Delphi survey, and doctors use it when they have a question that can't be answered by conventional means, usually because there's a lack of specific data. They ask experts for their recommendations, put the recommendations together, and then return several times and ask the experts again: "This is what your colleagues recommended: Would you change your mind? What would you do now?"

There was no consensus. Some said do nothing. Others said to give Beth isoniazid. Some said isoniazid and rifampin, or rifampin and pyrazinamide, or rifampin and ofloxacin. Most of the experts said that Beth should take at least two anti-TB drugs. Some said to take four drugs. One said, "Pray." The experts could not agree. I recommended that Beth take four drugs used to treat active TB, even though she only had latent TB infection.

She stuck to the regimen: "Eight pills a day. They were very large and hard to get down. I would gag when I tried to take them. The idea of not taking anything and hoping I wouldn't get sick was very appealing. I understood why patients don't comply with treatment. I realized how ridiculous it was to send them home and tell them to take maybe 15 pills a day." Beth took the pills at night, so as to sleep through the side effects. It was a difficult time, because she was an intern, working long hours.

Ten years later, Beth remains healthy. She hopes that the drugs she took killed off any TB bacteria in her system. She completed her training in cardiology, worked with the Indian Health Service in the Southwest, where TB is relatively common, and is now a practicing cardiologist in Arizona. She will always be more alert for any patient with weight loss, night sweats, and a lingering cough.

And Merlande, the little Haitian girl? She died.

Déjà Vu All Over Again

New York's epidemic wasn't contained just with money. Just as important was organization, something that the New Yorkers did very well and something that I've been trying to impress the need for on my Russian colleagues. The Russian system of organization was a structure of hospitals, sanatoriums, dispensaries, doctors, nurses, and technicians. It wasn't good at keeping track of patients, seeing that they completed treatment and finding them if they didn't keep appointments, keeping meticulous records on every single patient, and reviewing the records frequently. In Russia, if the patients didn't come back, well, they fell through the cracks.

At my medical center, teams met each week to review records and each outreach worker was personally responsible for following up with patients. In our New Jersey program and in some programs elsewhere, case management was the key. No patient escaped the system. The outreach worker watched every patient take every pill and recorded it. Every patient's record was reviewed every week. If a patient somehow went missing, it was the responsibility of the outreach worker to locate the patient. Accountability was essential, and dedicated outreach workers did the job. In 1989, fewer than half of all New York TB patients had completed treatment. By 1994, 90 percent of all patients completed treatment.

Controlling New York's epidemic was expensive, but far cheaper than hospitalizing patients desperately ill with tuberculosis and those they had infected. It's wrong to say, as many do, that it cost $1 billion. Dr. Hamburg stressed that the correct view is that the epidemic cost New York City $1 billion in excess health costs that could have been avoided if TB had been treated effectively in the first place. It is, she said, "A case of pay now or pay later."

When the epidemic was over, Hamburg said she felt fortunate about how it had been handled. "I never thought we could make as big a difference as we did, given the time frame we had. There was an astounding decline in multi-drug-resistant TB cases—91 percent." The TB rate in New York City is now down to 16.6 cases per 100,000, much lower than it was before the epidemic. This is still almost three times the national rate of 5.8 per 100,000, but both are far above the national goal, which had been set at 3.5 cases per million for the year 2000. In other words, a chance was lost, then regained at great cost and with the help of dedicated public health workers, and New York in 2000 was finally below where it had started from, about 20 years before.

Dr. Paula Fujiwara took over as head of the Bureau of Tuberculosis Control at New York City's Department of Health after Frieden left to work against TB in India with the World Health Organization. With the continuing progress in New York City, Fujiwara moved on, too. In 2001 she moved to the International Union Against Tuberculosis and Lung Disease, in Paris, the major nongovernmental organization that has been fighting TB internationally since 1920. She became deputy executive director, where the organizational and diplomatic skills she demonstrated in New York will be invaluable in fighting TB and multi-drug-resistant TB on a global level.

Just before she left New York, Fujiwara considered the current situation in the city. She sighed. Her budget had been cut again. "It's not a crisis any more, and when it's not a crisis it's hard to get people interested. It's my responsibility to keep TB in the forefront. You do have to have vigilance to prevent it coming back. I've actually heard some people argue that it would cost less to ignore TB now and just reinvest the money when it gets bad again. They say, 'You got it under control once, so you can do it again.'"

10

DOTS in the Real World

Rebecca Stevens is one of the unsung heroes in the campaign against TB. She is an outreach worker on one of the three outreach teams at the New Jersey Medical School National Tuberculosis Center in Newark. "I wore high heels and a suit every day before I came to this job," Stevens told Janice Tanne. "Before, I was office manager for a tableware firm. It took me 3 days to change my dress code. I was begging to be mugged. I wasn't there to impress people. I realized I'm here to do my job, not to do my job and die. I bought my first pair of sneakers since high school. I get my jeans from my nephew. People give me T-shirts."

Beneath those baggy, nondescript clothes, Stevens was a slim, attractive African American woman in her forties who must have looked very professional when her business attire was high heels and a suit. In baggy jeans, a faded T-shirt, and sneakers, she blended more easily into the community she serves. She had a cheerful, friendly manner, rather like a big sister. Perhaps it came from having grown up in a big family on a farm in the South, though she and her husband now lived in Newark.

As an outreach worker, Rebecca Stevens treated people in the community who had active tuberculosis, making sure they took their many antibiotic pills on schedule. Her work prevented her patients from dying from tuberculosis and protected their children, other people in their households, and their schoolmates and neighbors from becoming infected. It also protected everyone who rode the bus or subway with her patients or went to the same school, movie theater, church, or community center.

Her work helped to prevent a future epidemic from erupting in the community. She treated people who had latent TB infection to prevent them from getting sick in the future. She also did contact investigation: She interviewed patients, tracked down people whom they might have infected, and referred those people for evaluation. "Contacts" included people who lived in the same household, people who worked or went to school with the patient, close friends, and, as we saw when we investigated the outbreak in the church choir (see Chapter 8, "Fingerprinting the Bacteria"), people who shared community activities.

Until the 1960s, Newark was a prosperous city, with railroads, harbor, and manufacturing industries. It was a middle-class city, with headquarters of insurance firms, a major shopping district with big department stores, and excellent transportation—which still remains—to New York and to all the cities up and down the East Coast corridor from Boston to Washington. In 1967, riots that followed the beating of a black cab driver by white police officers destroyed much of the downtown business district. Ironically, one underlying reason that the riots erupted was the planned building of my medical center in the Central Ward of Newark. The University of Medicine and Dentistry of New Jersey would unfortunately displace about 1000 poor, mainly black people, who lived in the center of the Newark ghetto. After the riots, the university was built, but with an agreement that allowed for unprecedented community involvement in its governance and with promises of work for many minority individuals. Indeed, today the university is the largest employer, as well as the largest employer of minorities, in Newark.

After the riots, most of Newark's middle class, both white and black, left. What hadn't been burned down in the riots became dilapidated and either fell down or was bulldozed. There are still vast empty tracts, whole square blocks of earth and green weeds, with bare roads running through them. Once these were neighborhoods, not too grand, but busy, with shops and delicatessens and restaurants. There were buildings three or four stories high, with apartments above the shops. Small row houses lined the streets.

Today, rising above this wasteland are rows of huge red brick public housing projects, notorious for drugs and crime, that the city has begun to knock down. Things are getting better. Urban renewal projects and private investors are building small, attractive, two- and three-story townhouses on those bare acres, lining the streets with trees and the bicycles, tricycles, and barbecues of suburban-style life.

Downtown there are shiny mirror-glass office buildings, a law school, an extremely popular and successful new performing arts center, and a new minor league baseball stadium. Plans are underway for a major sports arena complex. Only 10 minutes from downtown is the busiest airport in the New York area.

The Directly Observed Therapy Rounds

When we started "case management"—which involves outreach workers such as Rebecca Stevens who are accountable to their supervisors and who make it easy for patients to complete TB treatment—our success rate soared from about 50 to 98 percent. The method has clearly saved the lives of many of our patients and protected their families, friends, and neighbors. Stevens and her colleagues were the key to our success through their persistence and their meticulous record keeping, which did not let patients fall through the cracks. Each day, Stevens started her rounds at a simple cubicle in the National TB Center's Lattimore Clinic. She picked up several white paper bags, each containing the medication she would deliver to a patient. She would watch each patient swallow the pills. As incentives to complete treatment, patients might also get $5 vouchers for the local transport system, $5 coupons for local supermarkets, or cans of nutritious drinks.

Stevens drove through her territory in her own car; she would be reimbursed for mileage. The territory included middle-class apartments in old one-family houses, small townhouses, and Newark's notorious high-rise public housing projects. On this particular day, her first stop was Joanne, a woman in her 20s. (Names and some personal details of patients in this chapter have been changed to protect their privacy.) Joanne had been treated at University Hospital for TB that she had probably caught from her boyfriend. She had been ill with what her local private doctor called pneumonia for 3 months. Although she had had a positive skin test for TB, she had never had a chest X-ray, the next most basic follow-up step. When it was recognized that she might have been infected with TB through her boyfriend, she took isoniazid, a preventive drug, for 2 months, but she stopped far short of the usual nine-month course of treatment for latent TB infection. Since her TB infection had not been treated appropriately, she ultimately needed hospitalization for what turned out to be active TB. When she left the hospital, she moved in with her mother, who lived in a big, old-fashioned, Archie Bunker-style house. Stevens's job was to make sure that Joanne now took the full treatment for tuberculosis. They met at the stairway leading to Joanne's apartment. Joanne took her pills and Stevens gave her a six-pack of the nutritious drink.

"Some clients sell it to buy drugs or whiskey or a sandwich. Others drink it for the nutrition," according to Stevens. The drink had a good reputation on the street for being high in nutrition. The $5 transportation vouchers and coupons for a local supermarket that we handed out to many patients might also be sold, traded, or used.

Some critics railed against our use of these incentives, although some similar programs actually paid patients *cash*. Our objective has always been to cure the patient, no matter what it took. Incentives kept people on their full prescribed course of treatment. Since that's what it took, we used incentives liberally. We wouldn't get the results we do without them.

Stevens's next stop was a private patient whose own doctor had recommended that he get directly observed therapy from our service because his TB treatment had failed before. Although this virtually assures cure, most private physicians still are very reluctant to avail themselves of the benefits of directly observed therapy. The patient lived with his fiancée and her son in a roomy, rambling apartment on the ground floor. Known simply as "Mr. MacIntosh," the patient insisted that he would see only Stevens. His TB was a reactivation of a previous episode of the disease. He had been taking the medications by himself, but when he stopped too soon, his TB came back. Mr. MacIntosh worked as a school bus driver. Since TB is a transmissible disease, all the kids who ride with him had to be skin-tested for TB. One child had previously had a positive skin test and had been treated in the past, so he's OK. One child's skin test had not yet been checked. None of the other children had converted their skin tests, so even though the man had pulmonary TB, he probably had not infected anybody yet. Even so, it was totally safe for the kids to continue to ride with Mr. MacIntosh because his TB would no longer be infectious, thanks to daily treatment, which usually makes patients noninfectious in a few weeks. However, he had to continue the medications until his TB had been cured.

Next Stevens drove on to find Charlie Atwood, an older man who shared a house with two other elderly men. She found one of his buddies, who told her that Charlie had gone to visit the clinic. She said she would catch up with him there.

About 90 percent of Stevens's clients did not have telephones, although they almost all had cable television. Lack of a telephone made it difficult for her to track them down if they were not home, and made it difficult for them to reach her if their plans had changed. Like a detective, Stevens spent a lot of her time looking for people. She found one client, who had been missing for 30 days, through the neighborhood mailman, who told her that he had moved around the corner from where he used to live.

Many of her clients had problems with drugs or alcohol, but Stevens made a point of not being judgmental about their lives. Sometimes she suggested that they not do drugs in front of their kids, but that was as far as she went. Her job was not to change the world, or even the neighborhood, but to make sure that her clients completed their TB treatment. Nevertheless, Stevens often became a family friend who was called upon to help with problems like a truant child, housing, or welfare benefits—almost a social worker. She was well known in her clients' neighborhoods because she visited almost every day for up to 2 years (to treat a patient with multi-drug-resistant TB), if necessary, and usually she was warmly welcomed.

If a patient would not answer the door, Stevens would return several times. If she still could not find the client, she reported the problem to her supervisor and the nurse case manager at the TB center. She continued trying the patient's home again, talked to neighbors and friends, and tried to track the patient down and persuade her or him to return to treatment. If the patient was a high risk to the community because she or he had active, infectious tuberculosis, the next and most drastic step was a stern letter from Newark's health officer directing the patient to comply with treatment. Often that worked, particularly when it was delivered by a health officer riding in a police car. If all else failed, the last step was getting a court order requiring the patient to be hospitalized to complete treatment. Diane Washington, R.N., assistant nurse manager at the National TB center, explained that our center tried to avoid the court order, relying on persuasion and encouragement whenever possible. Our outreach teams were set up so that there was somebody who spoke Spanish or Haitian Creole on each team. If a patient did not get along with one outreach worker, we assigned another—and another—until we got a good match.

Stevens's next client was a crack addict who lived on the top floor of a dilapidated building. Stevens rang and rang the bell and was almost ready to give up when the woman came downstairs, bleary-eyed and sleepy, although it was lunchtime. Stevens persuaded her to take her medication.

Jamal was next. He was a cute little 4-year-old in a spotless day-care center in an old church building. His skin test had turned positive after he was infected with tuberculosis by someone in his house. Fortunately, he had latent tuberculous infection, not active TB. Jamal needed medicine twice a week to prevent him from developing active TB from the bugs that he had caught. Jamal did not want to take his medicines, so Stevens mashed up the pills and stirred them into applesauce, which she then spooned into Jamal's mouth. He took it quite calmly and went back for his afternoon nap.

Like the other outreach workers, Stevens had 10 or 15 clients at a time, whom she saw 5 days a week. Next were two more of her difficult ones.

The first was a prostitute, so Stevens began looking for her on her corner. Across the street were derelict homes and apartment houses with young men sitting aimlessly but threateningly in front. There was no sign of the hooker, so Stevens parked her car and went into the only occupied building, where the hooker lived. It was a ramshackle three-story wooden apartment building with an intimidating dark staircase. Stevens started up the staircase, then froze at the sight of two huge, sleek, snarling dogs on the third-floor landing outside the woman's apartment. Carefully and slowly she backed down the staircase. Fortunately, the dogs didn't follow her. She knew that the woman's sister lived in a second-floor apartment. She banged on the door and gave her the sister's medication. Stevens warned her that she should not let the dogs out in the hall and said she would return later to check with her sister (the prostitute) about the medications, since all doses had to be directly observed by Stevens.

The next visit was no easier, but Stevens stopped on her way there to pick up a flavored pudding to treat one of her patients. The next family to be visited lived in one of Newark's notorious high-rise Prince Street housing projects. Fortunately the client, Susannah Lee, lived only on the third floor. Although some people would not enter the projects, Stevens did. However, she preferred to walk up the urine-stinking stairs rather than take one of the elevators.

Susannah was a young woman in her late twenties with three small children; she was Stevens's only patient with multi-drug-resistant TB. Susannah did not want to open the door to her apartment, but she finally did. Inside it was nighttime dark, as the blinds were drawn. Susannah became one of our TB patients 5 or 6 years ago, after she was misdiagnosed by a local physician. Even with sophisticated care in experienced medical centers, the cure rate for MDR-TB is closer to 50 to 70 percent than to the 98 percent rate for ordinary, drug-sensitive TB. Susannah was in and out of the hospital six or seven times with TB. Since her TB did not respond to drug treatment and she became severely ill, we did one of our very few extensive surgeries for TB. Surgery itself never cures TB. It may diminish the number of bacteria, but by removing some healthy lung tissue it may also diminish the lung's functional reserve if the tuberculosis relapses. That is why directly observed therapy is critical in postsurgery treatment. Now Susannah was receiving directly observed therapy with second-line drugs to make sure her TB was cured.

Her older daughter, whose skin test was negative for TB, got treatment to prevent infection, since she was in a household with a multi-drug-resistant TB patient. Her younger daughter had had active TB, but was treated and is now OK. Her son, now aged 2, was negative for TB as an infant, but his skin test became positive when he was 6 months old. Rebecca fed him the pudding she had picked up earlier, now with TB drugs crushed into it. Since he presumably had been infected by his mother, who had MDR-TB, he had to be treated for his latent infection with the same second-line drugs that his mother is sensitive to. These second-line drugs are more toxic than drugs for ordinary TB, but we hope they will prevent this young boy from developing active TB.

Stevens made a few more stops, finding some patients and not finding others, but remembering that she had to go back to trace them all.

Finally, Stevens returned to our clinic for the boring but essential part of her duties: meticulous record keeping. Stevens had recorded every visit she had made to a client this day. So had the people on the other two teams. Once a week, each team sat down for a record review, identifying where the problems were and what needed to be done to seek out the people who had missed appointments. The aim was to ensure completion of treatment and to prevent TB that might otherwise have occurred, by investigating and treating people who were contacts of those with active TB.

Once a month the information was reported to the state health department. It was entered into the state's computerized TB database, which records every patient with tuberculosis. We also report patients who have completed treatment and are now symptom free.

This boring, repetitive, detailed reporting is just as important as visits by outreach workers to deliver treatment to patients. My Russian colleagues are usually astonished by our painstaking record keeping, reporting, and tracking of patients. It is an essential part of case management. Nothing like this exists in Russia, as far as I know. Furthermore, Russian health authorities cannot force treatment on patients who refuse treatment or drift away, even though these patients are walking timebombs in their communities. In the United States we learned our lessons from Typhoid Mary and from the sensitive way New York City handled TB patients who didn't want to be treated during its epidemic. Their rights were carefully protected with free legal services, but if they did not comply with treatment, after several less onerous steps, they could be confined in a hospital isolation room until they were no longer a danger to the community.

As described in Chapters 6, "Inside the Gulag," and 7, "The Russian Style of TB Treatment," DOTS is the brand name for the World Health Organization's comprehensive system of tuberculosis control, which we practice in Newark. DOTS is not just watching the patients take their pills. There are also four other essential elements. In industrialized nations these elements are taken for granted, but in developing nations they often don't exist, even though they are what makes the system work. These key elements are political will, or government commitment to controlling TB through a national program; diagnosis by microscopic examination of sputum in a good laboratory system; use of directly observed, standardized drug treatment regimens; a reliable supply of effective drugs; and an information system to monitor and record treatment outcomes.

Providing the complete DOTS package is usually not a problem in industrialized countries. Their governments see it as an important public health measure. However, the directly observed therapy part is applied with varying degrees of effectiveness, even such industrialized countries. But, as we keep seeing in countries such as Russia, it is very hard to initiate and maintain *the whole package*, which is critical to TB control.

People sometimes ask if there have been any incidents between our outreach workers and patients. The answer is no. Although I often say that our outreach workers go to places the cops wouldn't go, in almost 300,000 interactions with patients over several years, we have never had a violent episode. Khalil Sabu Rashidi, one of our outreach team leaders in Newark, believes that the reason for the lack of violence in such a seemingly dangerous job is the close and respectful relationship between the outreach worker and the patient. "We are their advocates for their medical conditions, and they advocate for us on the streets," he says.

When TB Is Neglected

We do our best to find patients with TB and give and maintain early and effective drug treatment, but sometimes the worst happens or is thrust upon us and we have to resort to a Russian-style solution.

Four o'clock on a Friday afternoon, particularly before a holiday weekend, is the danger time. If something horrendous is going to happen in medicine, that is when it happens. I was sitting in the reception area of my TB center, chatting with my secretary Jean Norwood and my colleague Dr. Bonita Mangura and looking forward to the weekend. The phone rang. I made the mistake of picking it up.

For weeks, said an infectious diseases doctor at a hospital way across the state, he had had a patient with multi-drug-resistant tuberculosis. Treatment wasn't working. He thought the patient, a woman in her thirties, was going to die. Her insurance was running out and he didn't know what to do about her TB, so he wanted to send her to our TB center. The order in which the referring physician gave his reasons probably reflected their importance to him: first insurance, then TB. He wanted to send her immediately, that very weekend.

The patient turned out to be Maria (not her real name). When we saw her, she looked older than her age. She had been abused as a child, had dropped out of school, had abused alcohol and drugs, and had been in and out of jail for minor crimes. When she was still a teenager hanging out with the wrong crowd, a doctor had diagnosed her with tuberculosis and found that, fortunately, her disease was susceptible to the four drugs commonly used to treat TB.

But Maria didn't always take her pills. She wasn't much concerned about her TB, regarding it as just another one of those hassles in life that wasn't a major priority. Sometimes she went off with a new guy. Sometimes she moved to another town or stayed with friends. Sometimes she was involved with drugs and couldn't be found by outreach workers. Sometimes she was jailed and the jails failed to provide her with medications, which not infrequently occurs. For all through those years when nobody was paying attention, Maria had probably infected friends, lovers, relatives, and other people in jail with her, including perhaps the guards, the lawyers who prosecuted or defended her, and the court personnel. Nobody knows how many, and it would be impossible to go back and find all the people she was in contact with.

Now, after years of neglect, Maria's tuberculosis had become resistant to the four first-line drugs used to treat TB. Worse yet, it had also developed resistance to two of the second-line drugs we use for resistant TB. She had a bad case of multi-drug-resistant TB.

That's why her doctor wanted to transfer her to University Hospital. Doctors politely call it "dumping." Many community and private hospitals refer difficult, expensive patients to a university medical center, hoping that the state or the federal government will pick up the bill. Medical centers like mine feel that we have a moral obligation to accept these patients. Such transfers seem to be infinitely more common when the patient doesn't have insurance or when the insurance is running out.

The administrators of my hospital were reluctant to accept Maria because they would have to argue with the state about the hundreds of thousands of dollars it would probably take to cure this woman. Because she didn't have insurance, the state would pay for her care out of a statewide pool covering indigent patients. The amount my medical center would be reimbursed would be far below what it would cost to treat Maria.

Several years ago I strongly suggested that my state, New Jersey, establish a two-to-four bed confinement facility for those very rare patients who don't comply with treatment. During its 1992 epidemic, New York City successfully used just such a center to confine the very few patients who refused all convenient, friendly attempts at treatment, but New Jersey still refuses to fund such a small confinement center. Health Department officials, worried that such funds would come from their budget, said it wasn't needed because only a few doctors had tried to send patients to such a center. Perhaps doctors knew that it was futile to try to send patients to a center that didn't exist. I am convinced that the lack of such a facility in New Jersey leads to transmission of TB and multi-drug-resistant TB, such as in Maria's case, and that the State Health Department continues to fail in its public health responsibility by not establishing one. But even without such a facility, we try to work under whatever constraints are necessary.

My colleagues and I didn't think that Maria was going to die, even if the folks at the other hospital did. It would have been nice if the other hospital had called at the beginning of their foolish attempts at treatment, when we could have given the doctors there good advice and helped cure this woman with effective drugs. As happens all too often, though, they had screwed up this patient's treatment, and now they were dumping her on us.

It was Friday. I insisted that they fax a letter guaranteeing that they would take Maria back for follow-up care after we had treated her. They promised to transfer her on Monday, when our hospital would be geared to accept her and put her in an isolation room. Out of the blue, Maria arrived on Sunday. My colleague Dr. Reynard McDonald, a nationally known expert in treating multi-drug-resistant TB, rushed in and immediately put Maria in an isolation room with negative air pressure and started her on all the drugs she was not resistant to.

The drugs McDonald administered were second-line drugs (since Maria was resistant to the first-line drugs), and they had nasty side effects. After 2 months in the isolation room (which was costing the hospital $600 a day), Maria was not happy. Who could blame her? Even with television and a telephone, her life was acutely boring. She wanted to sign herself out against medical advice—AMA, as we call it. We knew that she had not followed her prescribed treatment in the past—in fact, she had disappeared many times. That was how she got multi-drug-resistant tuberculosis in the first place.

We were so concerned that Maria would disappear once again that we got a restraining order from Newark's Health Officer. She was a danger to the community, a walking timebomb. She could spread multi-drug-resistant TB to her friends, neighbors, family, and possibly everyone she met on the bus or in the grocery store—as, very likely, she had in the past. The restraining order, a very unusual procedure, prevented Maria from leaving my hospital. At the hospital's expense, a guard stood outside the door to her isolation room 24 hours a day. She had to stay and take her medicines until she was cured. The order also specified the medical center to which she must be referred when she got out. We assumed that she would survive, although we were not quite sure yet.

At 8 o'clock on a Wednesday morning, we held our regular weekly conference. Dr. Paul Bolanowski and his surgical colleagues presented their views. The pulmonary experts, Drs. Bonita Mangura, Reynard McDonald, and myself, as well as visiting faculty members and several junior doctors and trainees, presented our views, as did our nurses and outreach workers. This was one of the rare cases for which everyone agreed that surgery was needed. Maria's left lung could not be saved. Surgery should be performed as soon as possible, preferably after intensive drug treatment had temporarily reduced the number of TB bacteria in her body and made her sputum negative for TB bacteria. This would mean less risk for everyone in the operating room. If we couldn't get Maria sputum-negative, we would still do the operation. It would just be more risky for the doctors, nurses, and staff. We explained to Maria that surgery was her best chance for survival. She would still need to be treated medically for 18 months to 2 years, but surgery would make the medical treatment more likely to succeed. She waffled about it for a while, but then she agreed.

Surgery for tuberculosis is extraordinarily rare in the United States. In my hospital, which treats most of the tuberculosis patients in New Jersey, a state with a population of 8 million and several poor metropolitan areas, we may do fewer than five lung surgeries a year. In Moscow, a metropolitan area with a population of 9 or 10 million, 500 surgeries a year are done at just one hospital, according to Dr. Vitaly Litvinov, head of the Moscow government's Scientific and Clinical Anti Tuberculosis Center.

Operating Room 7

At 8:20 A.M., Maria was brought to the operating room.

The whole surgical team—the thoracic (chest) surgeon, Paul Bolanowski, his two assistants, the anesthesiologist, and the operating room nurses—wore double masks. And not just any masks; these were special fit-tested masks to seal the face against airborne pathogens. Each mask was supposed to be sufficient protection against TB. Breathing through one mask would be difficult, hot, and stifling, but these health professionals wanted double protection from the multi-drug-resistant organisms in the woman lying on the operating table. They were planning to breathe through two of these very uncomfortable masks for the next 6 or 7 hours. They were very frightened of the multi-drug-resistant TB that Maria had in her lung, because it would inevitably be aerosolized by the cutting and sewing and would float in the air throughout the operating room.

Bolanowski was going to perform a particularly brutal operation for tuberculosis that is seldom needed in the United States. He was going to remove Maria's entire left lung. Only Maria's right lung was working. Her left, riddled with tuberculosis, had collapsed, and a cavity full of tuberculosis bacteria had broken through her left lung and spread the infection into the pleural cavity, the space between the lung and the chest wall. It was like cancer spreading. There was a real risk that the infection would invade her remaining healthy lung. Although Maria's sputum tests had finally become negative, her left lung was still full of pus harboring TB bacteria. Her diseased left lung was getting almost no blood flow compared to her right lung. There was no way we could save her left lung. There wasn't any healthy lung left to save. By cutting out the diseased lung, we hoped to remove the bulk of the pus and scarring and to reduce the chance of spread.

Bolanowski was a stocky, determined man with sandy gray hair, hazel eyes, and a mustache. He survived tuberculosis as a young man, and now he was one of the few surgeons in the country who was experienced in removing lungs full of potentially fatal TB bacteria. Bolanowski had booked the operating room for 6 ½ hours—a long time, twice as long as it takes to do a coronary artery bypass.

Dr. Shuaib Akhtar, the anesthesiologist, gave Maria medication to make her sleepy and slipped a pulse oximeter onto her right index finger. The device measured the oxygen in her blood and would give a signal if the level went too low. This was particularly important during the removal of a lung because the lungs transfer oxygen from the air into the bloodstream. Akhtar slid a bronchoscope through Maria's mouth and down into the windpipe and then into the bronchi, the passages leading to her two lungs. He placed a double-lumen endotracheal tube, a tube with two small tubes inside, into Maria's bronchi. One tube went into the left main bronchus, and the other into the right main bronchus, permitting the anesthesiologist to selectively deliver oxygen to one lung or the other during the operation. The team was afraid of transferring TB from the sick lung to the healthy one, since that would probably result in a fatal infection. They inserted an arterial line on the inside of Maria's wrist to monitor blood pressure. EKG leads were taped to her chest to monitor her heart. A catheter was threaded into her bladder.

The six doctors—Bolanowski, general surgeon Marcus Kissim, chest surgery fellow Kirit N. Patel, anesthesiologist Akhtar, and medical specialists, McDonald and Mangura from the National Tuberculosis Center—inspected the CAT scans and chest X-rays posted on light boxes on the operating room wall. It was clear that Maria's heart had been grotesquely pushed over to the left side of her chest because her healthy right lung had overexpanded to take over the work of her disease-ridden and shrunken left lung.

Maria, anesthetized, intubated, and monitored, was ready for surgery. Bolanowski said, "OK, you guys ready? Left side up!" They were ready, and they gently rolled Maria onto her right side, padding her legs and body. Her left arm was supported in a sling above her body so that the surgeons could reach her left side easily. There were two puncture marks on the left side of Maria's chest, below her breast, where tubes had been used to drain pus from her diseased left lung. Bolanowski traced the incision he planned to make, a curved line between Maria's ribs, below her breast. In some patients, the pleura (the membrane lining the chest cavity) is so scarred and thickened by tuberculosis that it is impossible to spread the ribs apart and the surgeon has to remove a rib. Bolanowski was not yet sure whether he would have to do this.

Maria's upper body was painted with Betadine, a brownish antiseptic that looks like dried blood, and then covered with sterile blue plastic drapes. On top of those went sterile blue cotton towels, leaving only a small opening through which Bolanowski would operate.

With a swooping motion, Bolanowski cut through Maria's skin between the fourth and fifth ribs. A smell of burning flesh rose up as Bolanowski and his assistants cauterized small blood vessels. The huge incision curved up toward Maria's shoulder in back, up toward her breastbone in front. It looked as if they were trying to cut her in half, from side to side.

Bolanowski slid his whole hand through the incision into Maria's chest. He would not have to remove a rib. Kissim and Patel inserted metal retractors to spread the ribs and hold back flesh and muscle. As they probed inward, the surgeons struck pus in the pleural space between the lung and the chest wall. Bolanowski asked the nurse for sponges, then used a suction device to remove the pus. He was ready to start cutting Maria's left lung out, but the blood for transfusion had not yet arrived. He refused to go further until the blood arrived. He was furious, and his fury is legendary. Soon the eight units of blood arrived and he could proceed. Eight units of blood are a lot; Maria's whole body probably contained about 11 units. Bolanowski hoped he wouldn't need them all, but he said, "She's going to bleed like a sink."

Bolanowski spread Maria's ribs even wider. To his colleagues he said, "Now you can see the apex [the top part of the left lung]. What we have to do is nit-pick our way through this mess. I can open this mess up just with my finger. You can feel where the hard parts are. See this caseous material?" Caseous material is a cheeselike substance that is full of pus and TB bacteria. Sometimes the caseous material hardens into a calcified mass. Patel accidentally hit a rough calcified area. It slashed through his glove and cut his finger. He left the operating room to clean his cut and put on new gloves.

In many ways, TB spreads like cancer. Bolanowski found unhealthy clusters of tuberculosis organisms around the important arteries in Maria's chest. Tuberculosis had also invaded many lymph glands in her chest. Much of the normal anatomy had disappeared. Bolanowski became an explorer in unknown territory.

Mangura and McDonald took tubes of serosanguinous fluid, a yellow-ish lymphlike fluid stained with blood, from the surgical field and sent it off for analysis of TB bacteria. Although TB is usually airborne, in a desperately ill patient like Maria it can spread through the blood and lymph fluid to cause disease elsewhere in the body. Meanwhile, Bolanowski and his assistants dissected down to the hilum, the major intersection where the lungs branch off from the trachea (or windpipe) and the great blood vessels (the pulmonary artery and the pulmonary vein) connect the heart to the lungs. Maria's TB might have spread to this critical area. The surgeons tied off the connections between Maria's destroyed lung and the hilar lymph nodes around it in hopes of preventing the disease from spreading.

Bolanowski cut out as many nodes as he could. They were bumpy, warty growths on the outside of the bronchus. He sent half of them to pathology, to be examined for signs of tuberculosis. The tests to be performed on Maria's lymph nodes were similar to the ones used to examine for the spread of cancer. The other half he sent to be cultured, to see if TB bacteria would grow from them.

Bolanowski and his assistants searched for the pulmonary vein, the pulmonary artery, and the bronchial artery, which shuttled blood between Maria's diseased left lung and her heart. These blood vessels had to be found, tied off, and cut before Maria's lung could be removed, or she would bleed to death in a few seconds. The blood vessels were almost impossible to locate in the disordered, diseased anatomy of Maria's chest, but Bolanowski finally found everything except the pulmonary vein and sealed them off. Then he clamped the bronchus, the airway that led down into Maria's diseased lung, and sewed it closed.

Bolanowski had not finished. He still needed to find the pulmonary vein. The surgery got tricky when he saw that Maria's diseased lung was stuck to both the pericardium, the cellophanelike tissue surrounding her heart, and the diaphragm, the strong muscle of breathing that separates the lungs and heart in the chest cavity from the abdomen below, by extensive scar tissue. Carefully Bolanowski and Kissim peeled and picked away at the scar tissue, separating veins and arteries, constantly suctioning away the bleeding that inevitably occurred. The pulmonary vein was not locked in the scar tissue around the pericardium, so they closed that. Finally they found the vein, "way the hell back," and tied it off.

Slowly and delicately, Bolanowski freed Maria's diseased lung from the chest cavity. When it was out, it looked small—a shrunken, ragged, shapeless piece of dark red tissue, almost like a piece of liver. A healthy lung looks like a lively pink sponge. He dropped it into a white plastic bucket filled with formalin, a preservative that would keep the tissue for pathologists but kill any lethal drug-resistant TB bacteria in it. The pathologists would still be able to see tuberculosis in the tissue, but would not be in danger of being infected by live TB bacteria. Separately, he took a piece of the pleura and sent it off to pathology. "I want to see how much disease they can find in this," he said. Pathology's findings would give a clue to Maria's future. Although the center of her disease, her left lung, had been removed, there were signs that her TB had spread—into the lymph nodes, for example. She would need antibiotic treatment with drugs to which her TB was sensitive for many months.

Now there was just a big red hole in Maria's left chest. Carefully Bolanowski and Patel brought the tissues together. They irrigated the cavity with warm sterile fluid containing bacitracin, an antibiotic, several times. They picked out a few more lymph nodes for testing. There was no sign of an air leak from the bronchus into the chest cavity, which showed that they had done a good job. Into the operating wound they injected rifampin, which they hoped would help kill some of the few remaining TB organisms (although, since she was resistant to this drug, it was probably a hopeful but not helpful gesture). Bolanowski injected a local anesthetic into Maria's ribs, because they would otherwise be excruciatingly painful when she awakened. He pulled the ribs and the muscles together and sewed them. Maria had a scar stretching halfway around her body. Because it was closed with surgical staples, it resembled a huge zipper.

As Bolanowski had anticipated, the surgery had been long and difficult. After nearly 6 hours, Patel and Kissim were finishing up, removing the monitoring equipment and the surgical drapes. Bolanowski was yelling on the phone to the nursing station. "This patient has multi-drug-resistant tuberculosis. She has to go in an isolation room! She can't stay here. We can't put her in the recovery room. Last time I did that there was hell to pay." Finally he got the word that the nurses would be ready to receive Maria in a negative-pressure isolation room.

Maria was in our hospital recovering from her operation for nearly 3 weeks. She was then discharged to her brother's home, a stable environment. She had a good chance for recovery, but she had to continue to religiously take the medicines to kill the TB bacteria still remaining in her body. With only one lung left, she would surely die if the multi-drug-resistant TB recurred. An outreach worker came to make sure she took her anti-TB medicines

We were terribly worried about compliance, knowing how often Maria had dropped out of treatment in the past. Then something remarkable happened: The power of the press. Her brother gave her a *New York Times*

Magazine article by Lisa Belkin about a young Vietnamese immigrant's desperate struggle with multi-drug-resistant tuberculosis and the major surgery he had undergone as a patient of Dr. Michael Iseman at National Jewish Medical and Research Center in Denver, just as she had done at University Hospital in Newark.[1] The young immigrant man in the article was still in fragile health. The story rang a bell. Doctors had been telling Maria for more than a decade that tuberculosis was a serious disease and that she needed to take her medications. At last she heard the message. "You mean this could happen to me if I don't take my medications? I might die?" she asked.

Overnight, Maria became one of our best patients. She took all her medicines. She was always there when the outreach worker came. As of February 2001, she had finished her prescribed course of arduous second-line medications for her multi-drug-resistant TB. She followed treatment to the last letter. It is very likely that she has been cured. As for those friends, acquaintances, jail mates, lovers, lawyers, guards, nurses, and doctors she met along the way, well, we can only hope for the best.

11

Why Are There No New Drugs or Vaccines for TB?

Drug companies don't really want to develop new drugs against tuberculosis, I argued during an international conference on tuberculosis sponsored by *Lancet*, a leading medical journal.[1] Just look at our experience with sparfloxacin, a very effective drug in the antibiotic family called fluroquinolones. It showed great promise against TB. In 1992, Parke-Davis, which held its license for TB development in the United States, sponsored a meeting of major TB investigators in the resort of Scottsdale, Arizona, to tell them about the exciting new drug and to plan trials to study its efficacy in treating tuberculosis. More than 40 different public health and academic groups eagerly attended. There was great excitement about the prospect of a new drug against TB—the first new drug in decades.

Unfortunately, that was the last we heard of the project for a year and a half. Then we learned from a cryptic letter that Parke-Davis and sparfloxacin were out of the TB drug business before they ever got in. Not stated in the letter was the fact that Dainippon, the Japanese drug company that held the world license for sparfloxacin, took back the U.S. license from Parke-Davis. The company did not want to position sparfloxacin in the market as a TB drug, because TB was a relatively small problem in industrialized countries. If sparfloxacin was first approved for use against tuberculosis, doctors would think of it as a TB drug and wouldn't think of prescribing it for more common conditions, such as bronchitis or pneumonia. From a marketing standpoint, it would be far more important and profitable to get sparfloxacin approved for treating bronchitis, pneumonia, and other conditions that are common in the industrialized world, where people or their health plans would pay for the drug. In a way, its approval for treating TB would be a kiss of death for the drug. Dr. Lawrence K. Altman, medical correspondent of the *New York Times*, among others, reported on the conference, and his front-page story in the *Times* partially attributed TB's global surge to drug companies' profit motives and lack of interest in developing drugs for TB.[2] The studies on sparfloxacin for tuberculosis were never done. While sparfloxacin has been licensed for treating many infections, it has never been approved for use against tuberculosis. Nevertheless, it is effective against tuberculosis, and doctors use it to treat TB patients who have multi-drug-resistant TB, in what is called "off-label" use.

Finding the Effective Drugs

The most important drug we have against tuberculosis was discovered nearly 40 years ago. One summer in the mid-1960s—the time of bikinis, Brigitte Bardot, the first James Bond movies, and suntans that weren't bad for you —Dr. Piero Sensi, a researcher at Lepetit Research Laboratories in Milan, asked his colleagues to bring back herbs, fungi, algae, and soil samples from wherever they went on vacation. Sensi was convinced that he could develop new drugs from natural products by fermentation. He was inspired by penicillin, which was developed from a mold that blew in through a window and messed up a culture plate at London's Saint Mary's Hospital in 1928. Dr. Alexander Fleming noticed that the mold killed bacteria on the culture plate, a discovery that led to penicillin.

One of Sensi's colleagues, Franco Parenti, brought back samples from his Mediterranean holiday on the French coast. One contained *Nocardia mediterranei*, a kind of bacteria. Sensi grew it in a broth and found that it produced a promising antibiotic with a broad spectrum of activity, especially against the mycobacteria family, to which tuberculosis belongs. He asked Parenti if there was anything special about his vacation, to help them name the antibiotic. Well, Parenti said, he and his wife had seen a terrific French movie about a bunch of bumbling bank robbers. And so the new antibiotic was named rifampin (also called rifampicin), after the film *Rififi*. It was the first of a class of antibiotics called rifamycins.

After the antibiotic from that sunny French beach was identified, researchers at Lepetit began the time-consuming, expensive steps to purify its effective component, test it in animals, and then, slowly and carefully, test it in human beings. Human testing occurs in three stages. Phase I and Phase II trials are conducted in a small number of healthy people and give the investigator information about how the drug works (for example, how quickly it is absorbed, how it is carried in the blood, and how it is excreted).

These trials also give the investigator information about the dosage level that is most effective for treating the condition without causing serious side effects. Phase III trials, the most lengthy and costly, involve larger numbers of people to determine whether the drug works in a large population and to detect adverse effects that weren't detected in the smaller previous trials. Phase III trials are often randomized, controlled clinical trials, a method invented in the 1940s (first used for the TB drug streptomycin). In such trials, the patients are usually assigned randomly either to the best existing treatment or to the new treatment, with neither doctor nor patient knowing which treatment is being given; this is called a double-blind trial. At the end of the trial, the results are "unblinded" and the results of the new treatment and the old treatment are compared to see which is better.

Sensi is revered in TB and pharmaceutical circles for his monumental work on Parenti's chance discovery. He developed an oral form of rifampin, making it more acceptable to patients than streptomycin, which must be injected. By the time the rifamycin family of drugs had been discovered, many strains of TB were already becoming resistant to streptomycin and other TB antibiotics.

Today the rifamycins are our most powerful weapons against tuberculosis. Rifampin is also marketed in two combination products: Rifamate (called Rifinah outside the United States), which combines rifampin with isoniazid, and Rifater, a combination of rifampin, isoniazid, and pyrazinamide. Convenient and effective four-drug combinations have been introduced in the developing world, but there are apparently no plans to get these licensed in the United States. Combination drugs—several medications in one pill—are a great help in treating patients. They make it *impossible* for the patient to skip one medication or another, leading to drug-resistant TB, because all the drugs are in the same pill. And, of course, a combined regimen is more convenient for the patient: Depending on the dose required, the patient needs to take only a few of the same type of pill instead of taking three or four different kinds. The rifampin molecule is also the basis of two exciting new drugs: rifapentine, which is very long-lasting and so needs to be given only once a week, and rifabutin, which is effective against TB and also against infections caused by difficult to treat unusual bacteria (called nontuberculous mycobacteria or atypical mycobacteria) in the mycobacteria family.

Rifampin was introduced in Europe in 1968 and in the United States in 1974, almost 10 years after Parenti had come back from his holiday with that interesting sample. This time frame for drug development is typical in the pharmaceutical industry. Thousands of potential drugs are tested, most of which never even make it to clinical trials. Only 1 in 200 makes it to the pharmacy shelf, but usually the industry must pay the costs associated with investigating all 200.

Since the 1970s, there has been no new class of drugs for treating TB. Indeed, we have been lucky to hold on to the rifamycin group of drugs. Lepetit Laboratories had a major, historic role in developing the rifamycin group of drugs. But Lepetit and its vitally important drugs were nearly swallowed up in a sea of corporate takeovers. Astonishing as it sounds, we almost lost these drugs. The company wanted to stop making them.

In the TB community, the hero of this story is Dr. Giorgio Roscigno, an impeccably dressed, dark-haired, multilingual doctor and pharmaceutical executive, who has a passionate feeling that people should not die of TB when treatments are available. "I was born in Africa, in Ethiopia. I was brought up there. I lived in Africa. I felt I belonged there," he told Janice. After medical training in Italy, Roscigno worked for an Italian corporation as a doctor in the Congo, southern Sudan, and Nigeria and then worked for Sudan's Ministry of Health. In his work, he saw hundreds of people die of tuberculosis.

When an Italian pharmaceutical company offered him a job as medical director for Africa, he saw it as an opportunity—"a different approach to the same problem. Nothing changed in my mind or my heart"—and he was able to keep his company involved in TB drugs through many years of five corporate mergers. He emphasized the TB drugs' importance and their role in preserving the company's image and reflecting the company's commitment to global public health.

His company, Lepetit, became part of the Dow Chemical Corporation, which acquired Richardson-Merrell and became Merrell Dow, which acquired Marion Laboratories and became Marion Merrell Dow, which merged with Hoechst Roussel and became Hoechst Marion Roussel, which finally merged with Rhône-Poulenc Rorer and today is called Aventis.

Mergers like these have been happening over and over again throughout the pharmaceutical industry for the last 20 years. In the last decade, the companies have become bigger and more global in their orientation. As a concerned member of the TB community, I have found myself dealing with new corporate executives almost every month, trying to explain to them the history of TB drug development and why their company's work was so critically important in the global effort against TB. When Marion Merrell Dow was headquartered in Kansas City, I made a point of flying out there to talk to what was then the newest set of higher-ups. Whether in face-to-face meetings or by phone or fax, I dealt with new people each time, people who had neither knowledge of nor interest in the company's distinguished history in developing TB drugs and were more and more concerned with the bottom line. Each new management team was more reluctant to continue work on the "unsexy" drugs in the rifamycin family.

Members of the TB community pleaded with drug companies, calling on their charity, benevolence, and good corporate citizenship to get them to stay involved in manufacturing TB drugs. We reminded them that it was good public relations to keep producing these drugs, if only to offset the bad publicity that invariably occurs when drugs have side effects or a drug has to be withdrawn from the market. Several times Aventis almost dropped the entire rifampin line of drugs, but ultimately it was convinced that it should continue to produce them, thanks in large part to Roscigno. Today, perhaps somewhat reluctantly, Aventis is the world's largest producer of anti-TB drugs, with about 17 percent of the market.[3]

Corporate concerns delayed the marketing of an important derivative of rifampin for many years. When rifampin was introduced in Europe in the late 1960s, the idea of short-course chemotherapy against TB—the treatment we use today—was just being introduced in drug trials conducted by the British Medical Research Council. A very long-acting form of rifampin, called rifapentine, had been developed at Lepetit. A long duration of action means that the drug can be taken at longer intervals, such as only once a week, which obviously makes it easier for the patient to stick with treatment, and easier and cheaper for health workers to provide it as directly observed therapy. The question arose whether testing of rifapentine should be speeded up so that the new drug could be included in the new short-course TB drug trials.

The Dow Chemical Company, which by then was Lepetit Laboratories' parent company, said "no!" The patent on rifampin still had years to run. The company apparently felt that it did not make sense for a pharmaceutical company to market two drugs that competed with each other. So rifapentine sat on the shelf for 20 more years.

If Roscigno, Parenti, Sensi, and many others hadn't fought the good fight, it is very likely that the rifamycin drugs would no longer be available and we would have a tuberculosis disaster worse than the one we have right now.

Rifapentine finally did come to market; it was approved by the U.S. Food and Drug Administration in 1998. In the early 1990s, the successor company (Hoechst Marion Roussel) had applied for consideration of rifapentine as an orphan drug and finally got it. An orphan drug is a drug for a disease that is so rare that there is no financial incentive for a company to develop and market the drug. TB, of course, isn't rare, but the term *orphan diseases* has come to be used loosely to describe diseases that are very common but that affect mostly poor people in the Third World.[4] In the United States, tuberculosis affected a relatively small number of people, and so rifapentine won approval as an orphan drug.[5]

Remember the Bottom Line

We may criticize drug companies for their seemingly uncharitable stance. However, pharmaceutical companies are public companies, owned by their shareholders and traded on major stock exchanges. Their earnings—or losses —are minutely watched by stock analysts. Such a company's first responsibility is to its shareholders. If the company doesn't report good earnings, its shareholders will dump the stock, making it hard for the company to raise additional funds that it can use for research and to compete for talented employees.

The cost of developing a new TB drug would be high, and the companies didn't think that the market was such that they would receive a sufficient return on their investment. Furthermore, there were existing drugs to treat TB, so why develop a new agent?

For pharmaceutical companies, the big, money-making drugs are those that treat conditions that are common in markets where consumers (or their health plans) are rich enough to pay. That means that drug companies concentrate on developing medicines for an aging, relatively prosperous population in industrialized countries: drugs for heart disease, cancer, diabetes, Alzheimer's disease, asthma, allergies, and impotence. The average cost of developing a drug from test tube to a prescription pill on a pharmacy shelf is thought to be $300 million to $500 million, so drug companies aim for blockbuster drugs that bring in $1 billion a year in peak sales.

Drug companies aren't interested in TB drugs because the vast majority of people with TB are young and poor and live in developing countries. Very often, neither the people nor their countries can afford TB drugs. Unfortunately, the TB drugs that are available in these countries are often sold over the counter without a prescription. Even worse, some TB drugs are sold in combination with a popular cough syrup or expectorant, so an individual with a cough might inadvertently take one of these drugs in the presence of active TB and create drug resistance. Many of these drugs are beyond their expiration date; undoubtedly some are fake. People who are desperate to get well or to help a family member may be able to buy only a few pills at a pharmacy, not knowing that a complex, four-drug regimen for 6 months is required to cure TB. They do not realize that their supposedly helpful efforts are actually contributing to the development of multi-drug-resistant TB and may be killing their loved one. Brief treatment of TB may make the patient feel well for a few weeks, but it will always fail to provide a cure, and very often lead to multi-drug-resistant TB that will be more expensive and difficult to treat—and perhaps incurable. Brief treatment may get the patient back to work for a few weeks, supporting his or her family, but when it leads to multi-drug-resistant TB that is a public health disaster.

Control of anti-TB drugs, so that they are used only in effective programs with good follow-up, is essential for controlling the epidemic. Although it sounds harsh, anti-TB drugs must be restricted so that they are used only in good programs. Otherwise, easy access to one drug or another will mean that more patients develop resistance and spread the TB to family, friends, colleagues, medical staff, and casual passers-by.

Is There a Market?

Might there not be a way to entice drug companies to enter the enormous market in the Third World, to the companies' benefit as well as humanity's? For a long time, the situation didn't look promising. In 1999, Diana Chang-Blanc of the World Health Organization surveyed drug company attitudes toward TB drug development for Stop TB, an initiative of the World Health Organization and other partner organizations. The replies to her survey were frank and revealing. The short answer: Companies weren't interested.[6]

The survey covered 19 drug companies. Only five of these companies were involved in TB research programs, a sign in itself of lack of interest in the world's leading infectious killer. Several companies said that they continued to routinely screen promising drugs to see if they are effective against mycobacteria like tuberculosis, but then they just store the drugs on their shelves.

The companies told Stop TB that TB research involved a high investment with limited commercial return. Furthermore, they said, TB was a difficult and dangerous bug to work with, demanding biosafety level 3 facilities. There was also a risk of patent violations if a company came up with a drug that was too similar to another company's drug.

Furthermore, the companies did not want a drug that was earmarked for TB and was not used for other, more lucrative, conditions. "You don't want a broad-spectrum antibiotic reserved for tuberculosis. It's the last thing a company wants," one executive said. Another commented, "If you're going to develop a broad-spectrum antibiotic, you want it to work against chest infections, urinary infections, meningitis." Only later would such an antibiotic also be used for TB.

Finally, companies said they didn't like working with governments. They claimed that doing clinical trials in Third World countries—where the patients were—would be difficult because of problems with follow-up: illiterate patients, no phones, and patients not returning for checkups.

The companies estimated the tuberculosis market to be perhaps $150 million a year, and they needed to generate sales of at least $200 million and preferably $350 million a year to justify the costs of developing a new drug. They saw little potential in the Third World, where most TB occurs. One executive told Stop TB: "All companies have limited resources. If you have to decide which drug to discover, you will try to choose those areas that provide a quick return because of less competition, high volume and price . . . where you can get your return back fast. You will be looking in cancer, hypertension, Alzheimer's, central nervous system. Tuberculosis . . . maybe somebody else will think about tuberculosis."

Also, they expected to be pressured by the World Health Organization and national governments to sell such drugs at a low price. If they did not do so, copycat drugs could be imported from countries that do not honor Western patents. "If these pirate companies . . . are allowed to thrive, there will never be research in tuberculosis," a pharmaceutical executive told Stop TB. Another executive held up as a distressing example the response to an altruistic action by Merck. "Merck earns $1 billion in sales [from ivermectin] as a dog heartworm product, which allows the company to give it away for river blindness," a devastating disease that affects people in Africa. "Now there is an expectation from WHO that companies have to give drugs for free."

Drug companies often sell a drug for higher prices in prosperous industrialized countries, thus subsidizing their sales of the same drug for lower prices in Third World countries. However, another executive pointed out that this strategy wouldn't work for TB drugs, because they could not be sold at very high prices in industrialized countries. Most patients in industrialized countries were poor and couldn't afford the drugs, so they were purchased by public health authorities, which had the clout to negotiate large volume discounts. "The market defines the price," says Roscigno. Even so, the four drugs used in standard TB treatment may cost about $900 for a full course of treatment in the United States but as little as $11 in developing countries.[7]

Furthermore, the companies said, why bother to develop new drugs for TB? The World Health Organization—perhaps with its characteristic hyperbole—had repeatedly told the TB community that its DOTS strategy using existing drugs was all the world needed to control TB. While it is true that the DOTS strategy cures 95 percent of patients when it is carefully administered, we still need better, more powerful drugs so that we don't need to treat patients for such a long time. We will also need new drugs as resistance to the existing drugs continues to increase.

"Tuberculosis is life-threatening, but it has no commercial value" is the way one drug company executive summed up the situation.

He may be wrong.

Things began to change when economists and social activists joined public health experts in looking at the TB situation and showed that the market for TB drugs was much larger than had previously been thought. The Rockefeller Foundation got involved and brought with it the Medical Research Council of South Africa, the Stop TB initiative of the World Health Organization, the U.S. National Institutes of Health, the Bill and Melinda Gates Foundation, the Wellcome Trust, and the U.K. Department of International Development. Dr. Ariel Pablos-Mendez, an energetic and enthusiastic consultant to the Rockefeller Foundation and an assistant professor at Columbia University's Mailman School of Public Health, was the driving force behind the Rockefeller initiative on TB.

On February 6, 2000, thin, intense Dr. Anthony Mbewu, executive director for research of the South African Medical Research Council, opened a remarkable meeting on developing new drugs for TB sponsored by the Rockefeller Foundation in Cape Town, South Africa. He said, "We know that it is 35 years since a truly new drug, rifampin, came on the market [against tuberculosis] . . . that the last time a new vaccine came onto the market was 80 years ago. We know that progress has been pitifully small in the world of TB research and TB control."[8] Speaking to more than 100 world TB experts in a hotel ballroom, Dr. Mbewu pointed out the rapid advances in developing drugs and a vaccine for AIDS, a new disease identified only in the last 20 years. His nation was suffering a devastating AIDS epidemic in which tuberculosis was the leading cause of death in AIDS-infected people.

At the same meeting, Dr. Sunil Chacko of the Rockefeller Foundation reported that the global market for TB drugs was probably much larger than the $300 to $350 million estimated by the pharmaceutical industry. That was only the private market. When you add in the money that governments spend to buy drugs to treat their citizens and the fact that the market for TB drugs is growing by 8 or 9 percent a year, the market will probably be at least $700 million by 2008. Furthermore, if a revolutionary new drug appeared that could dramatically shorten treatment, it would almost immediately command a market of $300 million to $400 million a year.

Those numbers were big enough to lead drug companies to take a second look.[9] As John Horton of Smith Kline Beecham International said, you cannot browbeat industry. You have to provide it with facts and data.[10]

Roscigno thought there were ways to encourage pharmaceutical companies to work on new drugs for TB or to make existing drugs available at lower cost. For example, a Western drug company that produced a new TB drug or allowed a Third World pharmaceutical manufacturer to make cheap generic copies of its TB drugs could be rewarded by having the patent life of a different drug that is popular and lucrative in industrialized countries extended.

Another approach would be for a consortium of private and public groups—a drug company and a health authority—to work together to share the cost of developing a new drug. In fact, that was what happened. Out of the Cape Town meeting came plans for the nonprofit Global Alliance for TB Drug Development. It was set up in October 2000 to give financial support to researchers and biotech companies that are developing new diagnostic drugs and tests for TB. It would operate in concert with the Stop TB partnership of the World Health Organization.

By April 2001, the alliance had received $40 million from the Bill and Melinda Gates Foundation, the Rockefeller Foundation, and other private foundations and was supported by some of the most important organizations in the tuberculosis field. The alliance's first request for letters of intent for proposals to develop new TB drugs garnered 114, of which 24 were asked to submit full proposals, and 5 or 6 were recommended to the full Global Alliance board of directors for funding.

Already two drug companies, Eli Lilly and Jacobus Pharmaceuticals, have announced that they would cut prices on expensive second-line drugs, those needed by people with multi-drug-resistant TB. That was good news, but the price reductions covered only a very limited quantity of drugs. There was the possibility of allowing generic drug manufacturers to copy some of the drugs, but since the drugs had such unpleasant side effects, no generic manufacturer was interested.

At about the same time, the World Health Organization's Stop TB partnership, now under new leadership, set up the Global Drug Facility to buy and supply good-quality, effective drugs to nations with major TB problems. The facility would not manufacture the drugs itself, but would buy them from reputable suppliers. The drugs would be sold at low cost or made available free, but only to those countries that agreed to use them responsibly.

This means a system of DOTS, which, by definition, includes good reporting, record keeping, and follow-up. Initial funding was provided by the government of Canada, and negotiations that are likely to lead to awards were held with Kenya, Moldova, Myanmar, Somalia, and Tajikistan.

For me and all of the "usual suspects" in the TB community, seeing these new, extremely powerful players involved in the development of meaningful and practical programs was hopeful news. They finally had recognized that TB was a global problem, and they had new ideas and new money for combating this ancient disease. We found ourselves at a crossroads of global TB control. Perhaps we would take the high road to the sunny uplands of health and prosperity for all.

Or maybe we wouldn't—but that story came later, with the continuing, difficult, stalling, on-and-off negotiations for the World Bank loan to Russia, and in what I was seeing around the world's other TB hot spots.

The New World of the TB Genome

While we had made progress in providing inexpensive, reliable supplies of today's TB drugs to well-designed treatment programs, we knew that we needed better drugs that would allow shorter periods of treatment. If treatment of TB could be shortened from 6 months to 2 months or less, patients would be more likely to complete their treatment and there would be great savings for them, their families, and their nations. They would go back to work sooner, and health costs would drop.

Breakthroughs in understanding tuberculosis bacteria will come from new genetic knowledge that will show us new approaches to drugs and vaccines against the disease. The tuberculosis genome, all the genes that tell the bug how to live and how to kill humans, has been sequenced, or decoded. With about 4000 genes, it is much smaller than the human genome, which has about 30,000. Within years, or perhaps a few decades, we will learn how the genes work. In ways that are still mysterious, the genes of the TB bug provide instructions for making proteins that are essential for its survival and for its ability to infect us. When we know what those proteins are, we can develop drugs or vaccines that target them.

Two versions of the TB genome have recently been sequenced. In 1998, a team from the Sanger Centre in Cambridge in Britain and one at the Pasteur Institute in Paris sequenced the genes for an old virulent strain (H37Rv) that had been studied in laboratories since 1905. Another team, at The Institute for Genomic Research (TIGR) in the United States, soon sequenced a different virulent strain (CDC1551, sometimes called the

Oshkosh strain), the one that infected Charlie and caused the outbreak in the clothing factory on the Kentucky-Tennessee border described in Chapter 8, "Fingerprinting the Bacteria."[11]

The two strains differ in 1 of 5000 base pairs. These differences should give researchers clues about what makes a TB strain very infectious or relatively benign.

From the TB genome, we may also begin to understand the greatest mystery of tuberculosis: what researchers call latency, dormancy, or chronic infection. Consider these two common situations.

Most people who are infected with tuberculosis somehow control the TB infection in their bodies. It remains quiet, latent, or dormant until, in perhaps 10 percent of cases, it breaks forth into active disease when the person's immune system is weakened by age or illness. Of course, among people infected with HIV/AIDS, the risk is far higher: about 10 percent per year, not per lifetime.

Then there are people who have had active tuberculosis and have been appropriately treated. There are no more bacteria in their sputum. They feel well. By Western standards, by the World Health Organization's standards, they are cured. Such successfully treated people almost never develop tuberculosis again. However, they may have scars in their lungs from healed TB. Those who live in Russia often have to undergo major lung surgery to remove those scars before they can go back to work. Few Western doctors believe that the scars can do any harm; we think any bacteria in them are probably dead. Such patients, if they have been appropriately treated, almost never relapse; only the scar remains. However, Dr. Mikhail Perelman, the chest surgeon who is the head TB doctor of the Ministry of Health of the Russian Federation, reflecting what is surely a minority view, reports that he can grow tuberculosis bacteria from these "healed" scars.

So what is going on? Are there live bacteria in the lungs of people who were infected but never became sick? Are the bacteria multiplying? Are there live bacteria in the lungs of people who were successfully treated? If there are live bacteria in the scars, how is the body's immune system keeping the bugs in check? What TB experts call latency, dormancy, or chronic disease is a great mystery. If we solve it, we may be able to develop better treatments.

One of the reasons TB is so difficult to treat and cure is that TB bacteria are hard to kill. Aside from their hard waxy coat, which is difficult for antibiotics to penetrate, and their sluggish multiplication rate, TB bacteria have the ability to go into a state rather like hibernation when they are attacked by drugs. Drugs kill some TB bacteria quickly, but the bacteria that survive decrease their already slow growth rate. They reduce their oxygen consumption as well. Bacteria that are multiplying are usually the best targets for antibiotics. What's going on with these hibernating bacteria? Are the dead bacteria in healed scars really dead? Could they be present, but so disabled by antibiotics that they couldn't harm anyone?

No one knows for sure. We believe, based on our experience and many years of studies, that when TB bacteria have been so reduced in number and in strength by antibiotics plus the body's own immune attack, the immune system can then keep them in check. Recently, scientists have suggested that hibernating TB bacteria have a unique enzyme called isocitrate lyase that allows them to survive while other bacteria that don't have this enzyme are destroyed by the body's immune system. If they're right, that enzyme would be a target for a drug that would eliminate hibernating TB.[12]

So what triggers latent TB bacteria to wake up and run rampant again? Why does someone who was infected with TB as a teenager but whose body has suppressed it suddenly develop TB when she's 85 and has heart disease, cancer, and other problems? The answer probably lies in the way the body's immune system works. So far, we don't have a good animal model for the way tuberculosis behaves in human beings. All the animal models we have show a low level of chronic, ongoing infection, not the on-off-on situation we see in people. We have hints, but no answers. This remains fertile ground for immunologists.

Is a Vaccine the Answer?

Most TB experts think the only way to eliminate tuberculosis from the world is with an effective vaccine. They look to the eradication of smallpox as their model. Smallpox has been eliminated everywhere in the world by a vaccine developed in 1796 and an incredible effort by Dr. Donald Henderson and the World Health Organization. At first WHO tried to vaccinate everyone in the world, but that approach was clearly impractical. Instead, it identified outbreaks of smallpox, isolated the patients, and vaccinated all their contacts in a ripple sort of approach, preventing the spread of the infection. The method succeeded: The last case of smallpox occurred in Somalia in 1977.

Developing an effective vaccine that provides lifelong protection against TB infection is going to take a long time. Even if we find a promising, safe vaccine, it will take years to see whether it gives long-lasting protection to patients.[13] We would have to keep track of millions of people all over the world for their whole lives to know for sure.

A vaccine that prevents infection by a disease, like the one against small-pox, is called a prophylactic vaccine. We are fortunate today to have such vaccines against many diseases, such as polio, measles, mumps, rubella, and other killers of children and young adults. A *prophylactic vaccine* challenges the body's immune system by presenting it with a substance that is related to the disease microbe but harmless. This may be a dead microbe or one that has been weakened so that it can't cause disease. If the person later meets up with the disease-causing virus or bacteria, the immune system rec-ognizes the virus or bacteria and destroys it. Ideally, a tuberculosis vaccine would be given to babies at birth and would prevent them from ever get-ting TB during their lives.

However, vaccine researchers are looking for a quicker approach, called a therapeutic vaccine. A *therapeutic vaccine* protects against a disease *after* the person has been infected. In all of human history, only one such vaccine has ever been developed, the one that Pasteur created 120 years ago to pro-tect against rabies after infection.

An ideal TB vaccine would combine the prophylactic and therapeutic approaches. It would protect a baby against becoming infected with tuber-culosis, but if the baby did become infected, it would also protect the baby against developing tuberculosis disease during its entire life. It would require only one dose and would be given orally rather than by injection. It would have no side effects. Furthermore, the vaccine would not confuse the TB skin test, as the nearly useless BCG vaccination does. (However, if everyone were to be vaccinated and the vaccine was highly effective, we probably wouldn't even need the tuberculin skin test anymore, so the skin test status wouldn't matter.) An ideal vaccine would be cheap to manufacture and would be easy to transport and store (it wouldn't need refrigeration, for example). It would not interfere with other vaccines that are given to protect children, and it could easily be incorporated into the usual childhood immunization schedules.

Developing a broadly effective, long-term protective vaccine is going to take 20 to 50 years, but something promising may be ready for early test-ing in a year or two, according to two leaders in vaccine research, Carole Heilman, Ph.D., director of the Division of Microbiology and Infectious Diseases at the National Institute of Allergy and Infectious Disease, part of the U.S. National Institutes of Health, and Carol Nacy, Ph.D., director of the Sequella Foundation, who is betting her own and her foundation's money that it can be done.

Nacy is a vivacious and authoritative dynamo with an unusual blend of experience in the academic world and the pharmaceutical industry. She has worked in microbiology, immunology, and infectious diseases for 20 years as chief scientific officer of Anergen and Entremed, drug development consultant to Oncogene Science, and program director at the federal government's Walter Reed Army Institute of Research. When Entremed went public, Nacy took her money and set up a "small pharma" company to develop new technologies. And, in an extraordinary act of generosity and concern for public health, she set up the completely independent Sequella Global Tuberculosis Foundation.

"I never paid much attention to TB. I was one of the vast number of people in the United States who 'knew' we had cured TB worldwide," Nacy says. "In 1996, the National Institutes of Health asked me, as an immunologist, to help review the previous 5 years' funding in TB research and to project the goals for the next 5 years." When she heard the presentations of scientists who had been working in the field, Nacy was stunned. "I heard these outrageous statistics. The number of young people infected! The number one killer of women, more than any problem of pregnancy and childbirth! I was outraged by that. The number one killer of people with HIV. Number two killer of men. I realized how many people are dying of TB. We hadn't cured TB. We hadn't cured TB in the United States, and we certainly hadn't touched it abroad." She realized that there were many potentially compelling research projects in TB that needed funds for more development before they would reach a stage where they would be attractive to a pharmaceutical company. Among them were new diagnostic tools, drugs, and especially vaccines.

"Tuberculosis is such a complicated disease, and it's so dependent on [people having] intact immunologic systems that we could intervene in more than one place," Nacy says. "We're working on four vaccines right now, a better BCG, a replacement for BCG, a therapeutic vaccine to assist in and maybe shorten drug therapy, and another vaccine to prevent active disease in people who are already infected." She hopes that one or more of the therapeutic vaccines will be in early clinical trials by the end of 2001. The foundation is also funding research to find a piece of the tuberculosis bug that is recognized by the immune system in most people; such a protein could be developed into a vaccine. So promising is her approach that the Sequella Foundation received a $25 million grant from the Bill and Melinda Gates Foundation.

At the National Institute of Allergy and Infectious Diseases, both Heilman and her deputy, Dr. Ann Ginsberg, who is program officer for tuberculosis, have hopes for vaccines against TB. "We are close to early clinical trials for safety with one or two vaccines. We will probably begin in the next year or two," Ginsberg says. "It's not easy going," Heilman points out, however. "There is little pharmaceutical company interest. The big companies are waiting for small biotech companies or academia to come up with something."

Animal models of tuberculosis are not exact models of the way the disease behaves in humans. For example, BCG (vaccine) works well in small animals, but not in people. Efficacy trials will be long and expensive, the NIH experts say, and they will probably measure something other than disease as a marker of protection—perhaps a rise in certain substances in the blood (called a surrogate marker). These experts estimate that it will be 10 to 20 years before a therapeutic vaccine is brought to the market, and perhaps as long as half a century before a proven effective prophylactic vaccine is available.

Better Tests

We need fast, simple, cheap tests for TB, like the pregnancy tests you can buy in a drugstore that give yes-or-no results in a few minutes. The tests we have for TB are more than a century old and are not very accurate. For example, if a patient coughs up only a small amount of sputum or if the patient has only a few TB bacteria in the smear, a laboratory technician may miss the TB bacteria entirely. Tuberculin skin tests may be misinterpreted or may be confusing, even in healthy individuals, and commonly in a person with HIV infection. Chest X-rays often won't show early TB disease and never show latent TB infection.

Better tests may be available for use in hospitals and clinics in the next 2 or 3 years. Heilman's institute and many other organizations, including the Public Health Research Institute, are looking at new diagnostic tests in hopes of detecting TB faster and more accurately than we do now. Several tests look promising. One is a breath detector that spots patterns of chemicals unique to TB infection. Another is a "firefly luminescence" test developed at Albert Einstein College of Medicine in New York. Using a low-tech system called the Bronx Box, because Einstein is in the Bronx, New York, and luciferin, the "light up" factor from fireflies, it can show whether TB bacteria are growing in a sputum culture within a day or two, rather than in 3 weeks.

Dr. Fred Russell Kramer, a big, friendly molecular biologist at the Public Health Research Institute, bursts with enthusiasm about molecular beacons as another promising test. He is working with Dr. David Alland of Albert Einstein College of Medicine on this sensitive, fast way to detect whether drug-resistant TB bacteria are present in a sputum sample. The science behind the test, developed in only the last decade, is impressive. The result: molecular beacons, quickly cultured with TB bacteria, light up if they bind to regions in the TB bacteria that are sensitive to rifampin. In other words, if the beacon lights up, it says, "Shoot me. I'll die if you give me rifampin." If it doesn't light up, the TB bacteria are not sensitive to rifampin. Since TB bacteria that are resistant to rifampin are very often also resistant to isoniazid, this quick test could tell a doctor at a very early point in treatment, whether a patient has regular TB and can be treated with standard first-line drugs (rifampin, isoniazid, pyrazinamide, and ethambutol) or has the dreaded multi-drug-resistant TB and requires more toxic second-line drugs.

Using molecular beacons to test for the presence of TB bacteria and for their resistance patterns has many advantages. First of all, the laboratory worker needs to handle the dangerous TB bacteria only once, when putting them into a test tube that is sealed and placed in a testing machine. The test is easily automated, so that highly trained laboratory personnel are not needed. And it's fast. Kramer expects that a laboratory could test a patient in the morning and know by the end of the day whether the patient has TB and, if so, what drugs will work to cure his or her disease—a vast improvement over the weeks that it currently takes us to get this information. Furthermore, the lab equipment needed to do the test is about the size of a computer terminal and would cost less than $10,000, which is cheap for lab equipment, especially when compared to the hours of time now expended by highly trained lab personnel and the equipment needed to culture TB bacteria.

Good News?

You would think that all this was good news: New scientists are involved in TB research, and there are promising new avenues that may lead to new diagnostic tests, new drugs, maybe even a vaccine one day. Ten years ago no one would have cared, except for a few dogged people concerned with international public health and infectious disease, most of whom felt they were crying in the wilderness.

But a vaccine for wide use is decades away. Meanwhile, the epidemic is racing ahead of us. As I keep repeating, one-third of the world's population is infected with TB. Each year, another 8.4 million people become ill with tuberculosis. Two to 3 million of them die but almost every one latently infects 10, 15, even 20 people first, creating a timebomb of future disease. This timebomb is usually forgotten by clinicians and policymakers alike. In other words, even if a miracle potion were suddenly available that would *stop* all TB transmission and thus all new latent infections overnight, each of the 2 billion people already infected would still have a 10 percent lifetime risk of developing active TB.

In 1991, multi-drug-resistant TB was present in 13 states of the United States and in New York City, which was then dealing with its epidemic. However, although New York City's mammoth effort to control multi-drug-resistant TB was successful, things got worse nationwide. By 1996, 42 states, New York City, and the District of Columbia were reporting multi-drug-resistant TB. Among the hot spots identified by the World Health Organization in 1999 are countries of the former Soviet Union, such as Estonia and Latvia; a province in China; the Ivory Coast in Africa; the Dominican Republic; Iran; two Russian oblasts, Tomsk and Ivanovo, and a state in India. Just think how many legal and illegal immigrants from these countries are now in Western countries! And just think, in our global society, how many more are contemplating coming!

12

The Unusual Suspects

"I cringed when I saw the newspaper headline, 'Killer TB on Subway,'" said Dr. Peggy Hamburg, remembering when she was New York City health commissioner in the early 1990s. She was battling a tuberculosis epidemic in the city that is the world's financial capital and also the major U.S. port of entry for immigrants, tourists, and business visitors. But, while she cringed, she quickly realized that the headline was finally bringing attention to a problem that until then had been ignored by everyone except the small community of TB doctors and public health people, whom I call the *usual* suspects. As described in Chapter 4, "TB in the Time of AIDS," the New York City tuberculosis epidemic became front-page news in major newspapers and the subject of cover stories in international newsmagazines and special television programs. The epidemic was a threat to the city's economy as well as to its health. It took $1 billion in excess health-care expenditures to control it.

Money talks, and the frightening publicity helped. Those involved were not just the usual suspects, such as doctors and lung associations, the World Health Organization, and the Centers for Disease Control and Prevention. New people—"*unusual* suspects"—became involved, both in the United States and internationally. For the very first time, these unusual suspects included economists, finance ministers, politicians, tourism executives, philanthropists, grass-roots activists, businesspeople, trade associations, unions, and educators.

Often their motives were different from those of health-care workers, who felt that sick people deserved to get well. Economists realized that a sickly workforce held back a nation's development. Ministers of tourism noted that tourists did not want to vacation in a country with a raging epidemic. Unions, trade associations, and professional groups such as the American Medical Association wanted their employees and members protected from danger in the workplace. Perceptive journalists saw headline stories. Educators realized that tuberculosis was a lesson in history and politics for their students.

Internationally, one of the earliest unusual suspects was George Soros, the financier and philanthropist. Hungarian by birth, a Holocaust survivor, Soros had come up the hard way before he made his billions. During 1992, he made major investments in the former Soviet Union to help support their scientists and keep them from defecting (described in Chapter 5, "Smoke and Mirrors in Moscow"). He also recognized the moral, ethical, philanthropic, and economic imperatives of dealing with Russia's catastrophic health situation. He provided millions of dollars to help Alex Goldfarb (certainly another unusual suspect) and the Public Health Research Institute start their projects against TB in Russian prisons.

After the collapse of the Soviet Union in 1991, Russia experienced a disastrous fall in life expectancy—something that had never happened before in any country in peacetime. Russians were living shorter lives. The population was falling by millions, and the nation had soaring TB rates.

In 1993 the World Health Organization declared TB a *global health emergency*. This was the only time it has ever taken such an action. In the United States, the Institute of Medicine had held a seminal conference on newly emerging infectious diseases—tuberculosis among them.[1] Perceptive journalists noticed. Pulitzer Prize winner Laurie Garrett of *Newsday* published a best-selling book, *The Coming Plague*.[2] Garrett later expanded her subject to *Betrayal of Trust*,[3] about the worldwide breakdown of public health. Others in the mainstream media, such as popular American investigative television programs, began paying attention to TB.

Unusual Suspects

On the political scene in the United States, the first unusual suspect who recognized tuberculosis as a global health threat was Ralph Nader, the well-known consumer advocate and perennial U.S. presidential candidate.

At a meeting in the mid-1990s, Nader found himself talking with Richard Bumgarner, a former World Bank executive on loan to the World Health Organization's Tuberculosis Programme. Bumgarner's task had been to bring a marketing culture to that staid organization. The result was WHO's increasingly successful DOTS strategy and later its Stop TB Partnership, although Bumgarner and his boss Dr. Arata Kochi ruffled many feathers (especially among *usual* suspects) along the way. Bumgarner amazed Nader by telling him of the staggering numbers of new, active, infectious tuberculosis cases—at least 8 million a year—and the 2 to 3 million deaths every year. When most people hear these numbers, they are momentarily stunned and then go back to their other interests. Nader was different. He immediately mobilized the group he had established, Princeton Project 55 (PP55), an organization of Princeton alumni from his class of 1955.

Nader had reasoned that his classmates were reaching retirement age and could serve as mentors and role models for current Princeton students and serve the public good at the same time. In 1997 Larry Geiter, who was then director of research at the TB Elimination Division of the U.S. Centers for Disease Control and Prevention, and I spoke to the group about the global tuberculosis disaster. They immediately recognized the seriousness of the situation. Probably they were the first outside the public health community to do so. Their subsequent interest and involvement and their prestige and contacts proved to be invaluable. Soon after, PP55 started a program, The PP55 Tuberculosis Initiative, staffed by bright and energetic recent Princeton graduates, to advocate for global tuberculosis control. After a year or two, the graduates usually go on to medical school and are replaced by other Princeton graduates, a cycle that has repeated itself, but the "graduates" retain a unique understanding of public health and TB, and they brought about lasting, and important, effects.

In Washington, one of the first converts was Senator Patrick Leahy of Vermont, then the ranking Democrat on the Senate Foreign Operations Subcommittee. His eloquence about the importance of tuberculosis around the world, promoted in the House of Representatives by Representatives Rodney Frelinghuysen of New Jersey and Sonny Callahan of Alabama, both Republicans, and Nancy Pelosi of California, a Democrat, led to legislation and funding of an increasingly major new mandate for the U.S. Agency for International Development (USAID) to get involved in programs to prevent and treat tuberculosis around the world (which for many years the organization had inexplicably ignored and resisted).

Soon we found even more unusual suspects in Congress who supported the cause of ending TB. Among the senators were Democrats Edward Kennedy of Massachusetts, appropriations chair; Barbara Boxer of California; Daniel K. Inouye of Hawaii; and Republicans Ted Stevens of Alaska, former appropriations chair; Gordon Smith of Oregon; Kay Bailey Hutchison of Texas; and Dr. Bill Frist of Tennessee. Key leaders in the House were Representatives Sherrod Brown, a Democrat from Ohio, and Connie Morella, a Republican from Maryland.

On World TB Day 2001, in response to the Institute of Medicine report, "Ending Neglect," Brown and Morella, with Representative Henry Waxman of California, a long-time friend of effective public health programs, and 34 cosponsors from both parties, introduced the Comprehensive Tuberculosis

Elimination Act of 2001. The act provided $528 million for CDC efforts to eliminate TB, including program enhancement, preventive services, training/capacity building, including $240 million for research at the National Institutes of Health, tripling the NIH TB research budget. A companion Stop TB Now Act of 2001 authorized $200 million for direct implementation and expansion of DOTS tuberculosis control programs in developing countries with a high incidence of TB. Funds were also authorized for the Global TB Drug Facility, which would provide TB drugs at low cost to poor countries that are implementing appropriate DOTS programs. This was amazing! Thanks to these unusual suspects who had finally noticed TB, funds for both domestic and global control of tuberculosis had actually been appropriated in amounts that had never been seen before, and were being authorized to be appropriated in what could be considered *staggering* but justifiable amounts by both Democrats and Republicans.

Ordinary Folks Involved

Legislation affecting tuberculosis programs was greatly aided by other unusual suspects, such as a grassroots citizens' advocacy organization called Results, which is dedicated to creating the political will to end hunger and the worst aspects of poverty. According to Joanne Carter, the group's legislative director, it began to work with TB because "TB is both a consequence of poverty and a cause of poverty and because a cheap, effective TB treatment—DOTS—was reaching less than one-quarter of people ill with the disease. TB remains a health issue even in developed countries because of the threat of multi-drug-resistant TB flooding in from the world's hot spots."

Results believes (and has proven by its successes with TB) that ordinary people can make a difference in the politics of their governments and the priorities of their societies. Volunteer members learn to speak powerfully about issues and use that ability to communicate effectively with elected officials, community leaders, and the news media. These volunteers develop relationships with their members of Congress and with the editorial boards of local newspapers.

Since 1995, Results volunteers have been working with members of Congress and their staffs and generating much media coverage. They played an important role in raising congressional funding for international TB control from virtually zero in the late 1990s to $60 million a year in 2001.

On the international scene, the major factor that made the current situation different from the past scores of failed TB projects and task forces was again that new people—unusual suspects—were paying attention to tuberculosis. Soros was followed by economists, finance ministers, and tourism executives who began to think of tuberculosis as a hindrance to development. In March 1997, the World Health Organization and its Stop TB partnership organized the "London Conference" to tackle this problem. It brought together high-level economic ministers, health ministers, and government officials from Jordan, India, Brazil, Indonesia, and other countries whose economic development was held back by tuberculosis.

It's the Economy, Stupid!

Economists and finance ministers from industrialized countries saw tuberculosis as a threat to their own prosperous economies. About 450,000 people, mostly from nations with high TB rates, were seeking asylum in the European Union every year; many others entered illegally.[4] The borders of the United States were being breached daily by illegal immigrants, most of whom also came from countries with high TB rates. About 660,000 legal immigrants enter the United States each year, and the number of illegal immigrants living in the United States is now estimated at 7.1 to 9 million people.[5] Dreadful events like the discovery of 58 dead illegal Chinese immigrants inside a truck at the port of Dover in the United Kingdom, the stranding of nearly 1000 illegal Kurdish immigrants on France's Mediterranean coast in February 2000, and Mexican immigrants dying in Arizona on the desert border with the United States in the summer of 2001 alarmed economists, financiers, and politicians as well as public health people.

The London Conference was a very promising start. By suggesting that TB was an *economic, development, and tourism problem*, rather than just a health problem, it led directly to the March 2000 Amsterdam Conference for Sustainable Development, where 20 of the countries with the worst TB epidemics came together to carefully consider the way tuberculosis was holding back their nations' development. Some of the people who came were the usual suspects, the TB and public health crowd. What was unique was that each country also sent ministers of finance and development. These unusual suspects saw TB from a totally different perspective. Dr. Peggy Hamburg, who had successfully controlled New York City's TB epidemic, was asked to describe for the Amsterdam Conference how she was able to accomplish this feat. Listeners surely considered what an out-of-control TB epidemic would have done to New York City's economy and to its role as a financial capital. By organizing and managing the effort that ended the 1992 New York TB disaster, Hamburg had not only done wonders for public health; she had also protected New York's economy.

At the Amsterdam conference, the ministers saw and acknowledged for the first time that TB was holding their nations back, just as they would be held back by lack of an international airport, an inadequate telecommunications system, bad roads, uneducated workers, rundown hotels, or erratic electricity.

Health: A Key to National Development

They were not alone. The World Bank, led by its visionary chief executive, James Wolfensohn, was also looking at disease as a handicap to national development. Christopher Murray, a medical economist at Harvard University and the World Bank, pointed out that treatment of tuberculosis was the most cost-effective health intervention.[6] The World Bank recognized the importance for national development of a healthy workforce in its report *Investing in Health,*[7] and it made loans to Tanzania, Malawi, India, and China to combat tuberculosis. From 1999 to 2001, its representatives, aided by the World Health Organization, spent months in long and difficult discussions trying to negotiate a $150 million loan to Russia to combat the epidemics in its prisons and spreading among its civilians. In March 2001, the negotiators thought an agreement had been reached, but signing was postponed. A key difficulty remained the official Russian approach to TB treatment, which stubbornly and persistently still did not agree with the World Health Organization's globally accepted method.

The G8 summit of major industrialized nations and Russia, meeting in Okinawa in the summer of 2000, focused on health and issued this rather obvious sounding, but late in arriving, statement: "Health is a key to prosperity. Good health contributes directly to economic growth while poor health drives poverty."[8] The Japanese government promised $3 billion during the next 3 years. Members of the European Union were considering adding further funds. Members of the summit meeting committed themselves to working with governments, the World Health Organization and other international groups, industrial giants such as pharmaceutical companies, nongovernmental organizations, academic institutions, and foundations. Their noble aim was to reduce tuberculosis deaths and infections by *one-half within 10 years,* and to reduce malaria and HIV/AIDS infections among young people.

Of course, governments would have to agree on the treatment protocols to be used. Drug manufacturers who could produce the large amounts of drugs needed would have to be found, and they would have to guarantee a steady supply for years. Local anti-TB programs would have to work out the problem of getting imported drugs through customs. International donors would need to work with the existing public health system. However well-funded and well-meaning any program was, it would certainly be a long time before it would actually reduce the number of TB cases.

In the United States, an increasing number of unusual suspects joined in the discussion. In April 2000, in response to a courageous request from the Tuberculosis Elimination Division of CDC, the eminent Institute of Medicine, part of the U.S. National Academy of Sciences, issued a comprehensive report on tuberculosis.[9] I call the request courageous because the essential aspect of IOM reports is their independence and objectivity. When Dr. Ken Castro, director, and Carl Schiffelbein, deputy director, of the TB Elimination Division, contracted for the report with the institute more than a year earlier, they had no idea what the outcome might be. The institute is no ordinary bureaucratic body. It enlists independent experts to examine policy issues relating to public health and to mince no words in what they say.

The title of the report, *Ending Neglect*, spoke volumes about the findings it contained. The report concluded that it was essential to continue the battle against TB even though rates in the United States were going down —not slack off as had happened in the 1970s and 1980s, leading directly to the increase in cases nationwide and to the New York City epidemic. It said that managed care health systems should pay for TB detection and treatment with directly observed therapy as a public health issue.

Testing Immigrants?

The debate is just beginning on one of the report's most controversial sections, which focused on the increasing numbers of U.S. TB patients who had been born in countries with a lot of TB, the so-called high-burden countries. Close to half the cases of TB in the United States occurred in immigrants. The report called for giving all immigrants from countries with high TB rates a tuberculin skin test to detect infection abroad, before they reached the United States. (Currently, immigrants must only have a clear chest X-ray taken within the last year.) Immigrants with a positive skin test would be required to *complete treatment* of their latent TB infection in the United States as a condition for receiving their "green cards," or legal residence permits. From an American point of view it sounded eminently reasonable to promote treatment of latent TB infection, one of CDC's major priorities. However, some European investigators were already preparing rebuttals charging the recommendations were not epidemiologically defensible and amounted to unwarranted coercion.

Similar conditions should be imposed on others who had latent TB infection but weren't sick, such as prison inmates, the report said. It called for tripling federal spending for new tests, new treatments, and a new vaccine, to $280 million. It said the United States should become more involved in global TB control and elimination. It called for mobilizing support to eliminate TB and regularly measuring how close we were to this goal.

Institute of Medicine reports are highly respected and widely discussed, and they get action and funding. The gist of the IOM message was: Now is our best chance to control TB and prevent disasters later in the millennium. The IOM report has led directly to introduction of new legislation that— when passed—will have a major effect in reducing global and domestic TB.

Around the time that the Institute of Medicine was preparing its report, another unusual suspect joined in the fight against TB: the Bill and Melinda Gates Foundation, set up by the richest man on Earth, Bill Gates of Microsoft. The Gates Foundation, advised by Dr. William Foege, former director of the Centers for Disease Control, made well-researched major donations to provide protective immunizations to children around the world and to support research on killer diseases such as tuberculosis and AIDS for which no effective vaccine exists. In mid-2000, the Gates Foundation gave a staggering $46 million to Dr. Paul Farmer and Dr. Jim Kim's Partners in Health organization, which had been successful in treating poor people with MDR-TB from one barrio in Lima, to reproduce its success on a countrywide scale in Peru using DOTS and DOTS-Plus.

Alex Goldfarb had also applied to the Gates Foundation for support for his Russian TB project and was bitterly disappointed at being turned down. Maybe that, together with another one of Goldfarb's amazing adventures, confirmed him in his decision to change course entirely, as I found out later.

Educating Future Leaders

Another unusual suspect is one of the most important of all because of its potential. I was delighted to learn about a grassroots effort to educate tomorrow's leaders about tuberculosis and the importance of public health. One day I got an unexpected phone call from a biology professor at Franklin and Marshall College in Lancaster, Pennsylvania, a small, distinguished school with pretty brick buildings set among lawns and old trees. Dick Fluck (pronounced "fluke") asked me if I would come and speak to his first-year student seminar course. At F&M, first-year students spend a whole semester focusing on a single topic. They learn how to do research, how to write a paper, and how to make presentations, skills that will serve them both in college and throughout their lives. Fluck decided that that topic this year would be tuberculosis.

He thought that the pre-med and biology majors would be interested in learning the new scientific findings about TB and the complex treatment regimens. Students who were going into law, politics, or social work would see the issues of private rights versus protection of the public from a contagious disease. Those destined for careers in public health or international business would learn that the world is a global village. In any case, the knowledge they gained would be important for them as concerned citizens, because they would learn that although tuberculosis is the world's leading infectious killer, it is preventable and curable largely by widely accepted techniques enhanced by an infusion of political will.

On a visit to the campus to observe the program in action and to participate in seminars with the entire class, I was impressed when these bright young people started talking about their research. They were smart, and they had obviously done their homework. I was certain that they knew more about tuberculosis than any other group of college students in the world, and far more than most doctors and policy makers.

I was heartened to have met these well-informed young people—a whole new group of unusual suspects—and really impressed by Fluck's zeal and passion in setting up and maintaining this unique seminar. I was even more pleased to observe and participate in the second edition of the same course the next year, educating another group of bright young people who can, perhaps, make the changes that have potential to eliminate tuberculosis from the world forever. And finally, I was delighted to learn that (with the help of Princeton Project 55) Fluck has just been appointed visiting professor at the Woodrow Wilson School of Public and International Policy of Princeton University, where that student body chose him to present *his* course as a senior seminar on their campus in the fall of 2001.

Perhaps Fluck has the right idea: Give the future leaders of our society a healthy fear of TB and knowledge of how it can be controlled if and when there is political will. They will know that the knowledge and technology to eliminate TB exist.

Political Will

"Building political will" is an awkward bureaucratic phrase that has joined the TB vernacular. It describes the essentials of getting the job done: recognizing the problem and agreeing on a course of action. Only just recently have public health experts come to realize that policy makers with political power must be made to understand that preventing and curing tuberculosis is vitally important, not only for world health but for their own national prosperity as well. When policy makers understand this critical point, we can then get doctors, scientists, and public health officials to agree on the best way to control TB in their nations.

The American Lung Association (the Christmas seal people) is America's oldest voluntary health association, known for its pioneering work in the successful fight against the tobacco industry and air pollution. It began as the National Association for the Study and Prevention of Tuberculosis almost a century ago, in 1904, although sometimes it has been difficult to sustain the involvement of its volunteers on TB issues when TB rates (and interest) were falling in the United States.

Fran DuMelle, the American Lung Association's executive vice president, senior policy person, and top lobbyist in Washington, DC, has worked for many years to develop political will on tuberculosis. DuMelle is an extraordinarily outspoken woman with a brilliant mind. I don't know if she plays chess, but she'd be good at it. She is very perceptive about how to move the various pieces and players. DuMelle recalls the important "London report" from the 1997 conference convened by the World Health Organization on ways to combat TB. "People at the meeting ran after policy people like me and said, 'Create the political will' without understanding what it takes to get to political will. That's Russia's problem today. The primary need is medical and scientific consensus. In the United States, we turned around the TB epidemic in the late 1980s and early 1990s with a strategic plan that everyone agreed on."

In the United States, the first attempt to control the TB epidemic was a mistake, according to DuMelle. The Centers for Disease Control wrote a strategic plan and presented it to the TB community. The TB community rudely rejected it. Actually, the CDC strategic plan as initially proposed and the plan that was finally adopted by the TB community were not that different.

"What you needed was a consensus," DuMelle explained.

"CDC recognized they needed everybody behind them in order to go forward. They went around the country. They had meetings. They spoke with the experts, asked what they were unhappy about. They used major organizations like the American Lung Association, the American Thoracic Society [the professional society of lung doctors], the American Public Health Association, the Infectious Disease Society of America, a number of organizations . . . to drag everybody kicking and screaming to a table and develop the elusive consensus. The leaders of the medical and public health community had to agree on what needed to be done. Otherwise they would each be fighting their own battle with the policy makers, who were already confused and therefore wouldn't do anything at all. A lot of the arguments related to how you found people with tuberculosis and those whom they might have infected. In the U.S., the treatment is pretty much standard, everybody does it this way. But in India, for example, most TB patients are treated in the private sector and one study found almost 100 different treatment regimens, and the overwhelming majority of them were absolutely wrong. When you get the initial treatment wrong, you are often well on the way to creating multi-drug-resistant TB.

"By the time the Secretary of Health and Human Services announced this strategic plan [agreed on by all the medical, scientific, and public health authorities in the United States] in '89, everyone was solidly behind it. I had a document I could go to Congress with and say, 'Here's the price tag.'"

Since the publication of the plan and its acceptance by key policy makers, congressional appropriations for TB control have multiplied, and consequently TB rates have decreased in the United States for 8 years in a row, and are well on their way to a decline for a ninth year.

No Consensus

In stark contrast, Russia was still nowhere near consensus on the best way to control TB with the money from the World Bank's proposed loan. Negotiations had been going on for 3 years and involved different views on how and where the money was to be spent and what treatment protocols were to be followed. The protocols were widely different.

The World Bank and the World Health Organization, its adviser, were negotiating with the Russian Ministry of Health, bastion of Priymak and Perelman's old Russian school of treatment, and the Ministry of Justice, where General Yalunin had a major TB problem in his overcrowded prisons. There were also representatives from the Khomenko institute, which endorsed the approach of the World Health Organization.

Political will, a consensus on the right way to proceed, was desperately needed but was not forthcoming. Meanwhile, the Public Health Research Institute's and MERLIN's model program against TB and multi-drug-resistant TB in Tomsk in Siberia could wait no longer. The situation was getting nasty, and they had to act.

13

Tiger at the Gates

The situation in Tomsk in Siberia was becoming critical. For more than a year, the Public Health Research Institute (PHRI) and the British organization MERLIN had been promising to treat prisoners with multi-drug-resistant TB who were isolated in the Tomsk TB colony, a regional center to which prisoners with active TB were sent. PHRI and MERLIN had promised to run a similar program for the civilian population with multi-drug-resistant TB, some of whom had caught multi-drug-resistant TB in prison—either as prisoners or as doctors and nurses. Neither program had started, and people were getting angry.

There were problems with importing effective second-line drugs for treating multi-drug-resistant TB. There were also problems in obtaining the approval of WHO's Green Light Committee; such approval would make getting a reliable supply of drugs to treat multi-drug-resistant TB easier and cheaper. Since multi-drug-resistant TB is invariably the result of people's actions, its presence in Tomsk demonstrated conclusively that the local program to cure ordinary TB had failed. Poor treatment of ordinary, drug-sensitive TB, even though it may be well meaning, almost always creates multi-drug-resistant TB, and poor treatment of multi-drug-resistant TB makes the problem far worse. In order to prevent just such creation and spread of human-made multi-drug-resistant TB, the World Health Organization set up its Green Light Committee process to evaluate any program's fitness to do the complicated and expensive treatment with second-line drugs (DOTS-Plus) that is necessary if multi-drug-resistant TB is to be cured.

According to Dr. Kitty Lambregts of the Netherlands, chair of the Green Light Committee, the Green Light process not only ensured the proper use of second-line drugs and provided them at favorable prices, but also supported further development of an evidence-based framework for treating MDR-TB, a framework that might be useful in future AIDS treatments.

To start such a program for its prisoners and get access to low-cost, effective drugs, the Tomsk project needed approval from the Green Light Committee. An application had been submitted, but the committee still saw several problems that it felt needed correcting before it gave its approval, which everyone agreed would ultimately be forthcoming.

But the oblast of Tomsk was not particularly understanding of this process and could not wait any longer. "The pressure to start civilian DOTS-Plus is insurmountable. If we delay any longer, we will lose political support in Tomsk," said Alex Goldfarb after a meeting with Tomsk Governor Viktor Kress. Governor Kress's support was crucial. He had recently been elected to the Presidium of the State Council, with direct access to Russia's president, Vladimir Putin. He now outranked the minister of health. Furthermore, because of Goldfarb's tutoring, he was the highest Russian elected official (if not one of the very few) who actually understood TB.

The situation in Tomsk was frightening. People working with MERLIN were being physically threatened by the relatives of prisoners and patients with MDR-TB. They were desperate to get their loved ones treated. It was a scary situation seldom seen in medicine: threats against doctors, nurses, and administrators who were doing their best to get things working in a dysfunctional system. Tomsk is a relatively small city. Many doctors and nurses are recognized on the streets, and patients know where they live.

Goldfarb, who knew how to get things done in Russia and how to get payments made through reliable Western sources, arranged for a steady supply of effective antibiotics even while awaiting the Green Light Committee's approval. "The drugs cost more than if we had had approval, but we couldn't wait," Goldfarb said. Not only did he obtain the drugs, but he also found a way to get them through Russian customs quickly, instead of having them stuck for months, as often happened to other Western importers.

On August 22, 2000, just days after the Kursk submarine disaster, when the nation was reeling with fears of fatal incompetence and regretting that it had turned down international offers of assistance to save the men trapped in the sunken submarine, Goldfarb, Farmer, and I flew to Tomsk on an aging Tupolev 154 of Siberian Air. There is only one way to get to Tomsk: Leave Moscow late at night from a dark and dreary airport, fly through four time zones in 4 hours on a crowded and dirty plane with smokers occupying the toilets, and arrive before dawn at the dim, two-story Tomsk air terminal. There, they are extremely thorough in checking to see that you've picked up the right bag—more thorough than in any airport I know of. And since our baggage included the first shipment of precious second-line drugs for the treatment of MDR-TB, we were worried about too much interest from the authorities. We sighed with relief when we got the antibiotics safely to our medical colleagues in Tomsk.

We didn't mind the hassles. We were thrilled. PHRI and MERLIN had finally inaugurated a project for treating multi-drug-resistant TB, and we were bringing the drugs. After drug-sensitivity testing, the first 31 prisoners in the Tomsk TB colony were started on the appropriate DOTS-Plus regimen for their multi-drug-resistant TB, along with four civilians, including a doctor and a lab technician who had almost certainly been infected on the job. The drugs we had brought, imported thanks to Goldfarb's finesse, would probably give these patients their only chance of surviving their disease. We hoped that good news of their treatment would reduce the threats of physical violence to workers in the project. Also, because Governor Kress had found funds to renovate a hospital building to be used for DOTS-Plus treatment of up to 300 civilian patients (including released prisoners who needed continuing treatment), the team hoped to provide continuity of treatment and thus a greatly improved cure rate.

In the early autumn sun, the wide Tom River was shining. To celebrate the inauguration of DOTS-Plus, we went out for a celebration on an excursion boat with the entire TB medical service of both the civilian and prison sectors, as well as many political leaders. The farms across the river were rich with their harvest bounty. Women were selling plump dark green watermelons along the highway. The elegant buildings of the university on the heights shone through the trees. We all felt like celebrating. Finally, we had done it. Done what? We had brought in precious second-line drugs, and thus had started 35 patients with deadly multi-drug-resistant TB on a treatment program that would give them their best chance of cure and a long life.

Of course, the Tomsk project adhered to the standard evidence-based regimen used in industrialized countries, and also, with great success, in many Third World countries. Alas, that regimen ran completely counter to the treatment approved by the Ministry of Health. It was being used in Tomsk only because the program had received a special exemption from Russian rules. On the boat ride, it was paradoxical that the doctors treating patients in Tomsk were excited and exhilarated by their new project, but they were also very afraid. What they were doing was certainly both medically and morally correct, but it might actually ruin their careers. They might incur professional sanctions, and worse, for going against the archaic and insupportable governmental TB rules.

There is still a lot of Soviet mentality in Russia. The rulers have changed; the mind-set has not.

It wasn't until 6 months later, on February 27, 2001, that WHO's Green Light Committee finally approved Tomsk for a reliable supply of cheap, effective drugs to treat multi-drug-resistant TB. By the end of May 2001, according to Dr. Alex Trusov who was managing the PHRI programs in Russia, the Tomsk medical team (many of whom had been trained in treating MDR-TB at our international TB training center in New Jersey) had a total of 58 patients in the long, complex treatment program. The patients included both prisoners and civilians, who were taking the arduous and toxic regimen to cure multi-drug-resistant TB. Second-line drugs are more toxic than those used in treating ordinary TB. They can produce many unpleasant but usually manageable side effects. Three patients had acute psychosis, a well-known complication of the medication cycloserine, and several patients had imbalances of electrolytes (important chemical substances in the blood) due to capreomycin. Only one patient died, of a heart attack unrelated to his multi-drug-resistant tuberculosis. Most patients had a good clinical response—they felt healthier—as well as good responses on bacteriological tests of their sputum and on chest X-rays. These outstanding results, with extraordinarily complex regimens, were greatly helped by frequent on-site visits and conference calls between the Tomsk physicians and their medical consultants at Farmer and Kim's Partners in Health in Boston.

It was a success, yes. It was working. At least in Tomsk, there was now effective treatment of multi-drug-resistant TB in both the prison and civilian sectors.

Who Gets the Loan Money?

At just about the same time—the autumn of 2000—and 2000 miles away, back in Moscow, the diplomats and the bureaucrats were still arguing over the proposed World Bank loan to combat TB and AIDS. The Russians had a huge TB problem and the fastest-growing AIDS epidemic in the world.

In the early 1990s in New York, it had taken $1 billion in excess health expenditures to control an epidemic that never exceeded 4000 cases per year. Even with the World Bank loan, Russia obviously had nowhere near that kind of money, and infinitely more cases! Russia's retired chief TB expert, Dr. Alexey Priymak, estimated that 2.5 million Russians have latent or active TB, are constantly exposed to someone with active TB, or suffer from complications related to past TB.[1] And 5 to 22 percent of them have multi-drug-resistant TB.[2]

In discussions about the World Bank loan, GUIN, the prison administration division of the Ministry of Justice, had the worst TB problem among the 1 million-plus prisoners in its Gulag. At any one time, almost 80 percent of all Russian TB patients and most multi-drug-resistant TB patients were in prison. Since they were held under controlled conditions in prison, they should be able to receive effective treatment with directly observed therapy, but, as we and other Western experts and journalists had seen in visits to SIZOs, prisons, and TB colonies, and had discussed with Russian TB experts, this usually didn't happen, nor was it about to.

Worse yet for public health was one of the frequent amnesties for prisoners with TB and those who had committed minor offenses. The amnesty released 140,000 prisoners in the spring and summer of 2000, with no clinical follow-up for their TB (or for any other condition), thus spreading TB into the community.

Since the prisons had the worst problem and were a threat to the rest of the population as prisoners were released, should they get the most money from the World Bank loan? The loan would be for $150 million and would cover both AIDS and tuberculosis. After many bureaucratic discussions, thousands of pages of memos, expensive hours of international phone calls, and a myriad of e-mails, it was informally agreed that $50 million would be spent on preventing and treating AIDS, and $100 million would be spent on TB. The prison health system run by the Ministry of Justice would get about half the TB loan, and the civilian health system, run by the Ministry of Health, would get about half.

Who Makes the Rules for Treatment?

Discussions went on and on over the method of TB treatment that the World Bank loan would pay for in Russia. The World Bank negotiators were advised by TB experts from the World Health Organization, which had been promoting DOTS around the world for many years with great success. A high-level working group, established by the World Health Organization and the Ministry of Health, had been meeting since 1999 to revise the Russian national TB policy. They hoped to come up with guidelines—a Prikaz or order—that would be followed by all Russian doctors.

Negotiators faced the different Russian rules. After Priymak's 1998 Prikaz 33 (Order 33, mandating that Russian doctors treat TB with individualized therapy, lengthy hospitalization, and frequent surgery), three other official—and contradictory—regulations had been published.

The first set of regulations, from the Khomenko institute, essentially agreed with WHO's recommendations on treating multi-drug-resistant TB and with the Green Light Committee's requirements. Since the rules had been developed by a leading Russian institute, they could not be regarded as foreign interference. The project in Tomsk was following these regulations, which agreed with international standards almost point for point.

The second set of recommendations, from the Priymak institute in Moscow, and the third set, from the St. Petersburg research institute of the Ministry of Health, parroted the traditional Russian approach to treating TB.

Ordinary Russian doctors, particularly those working with Western organizations, were in a quandary. Doctors at the Murmansk Regional TB Dispensary, in far northern Russia, who were getting help from a Finnish medical group, wrote an anonymous letter to the leading newspaper *Medical Gazette*.[3] They complained that their Finnish coworkers relied on bacteriology (examination of sputum under the microscope) for diagnosis, as do most enlightened practitioners in the world. That was different from the rules issued by Moscow. They suggested that their bosses were going along with Finnish colleagues so that they could get other, material assistance, such a computer and a fax machine. Were they to abandon traditional Russian ways of diagnosis and treatment?

The *Medical Gazette* asked Dr. Mikhail Perelman, Russia's top TB doctor and the adviser to the Ministry of Health, for comment. He said,

"The doctors from the Murmansk TB Dispensary are correct in their assessing the situation. The thing is, some head doctors, health managers, are easily bought. They will sell everything, including ideology and certain principles. In fact, for money you can buy disloyalty to the existing directives and orders coming from the Health Ministry, which is unacceptable. Since TB doctors work in Russia, it is their duty to obey our domestic guidelines and documentation. They are certainly free to discuss and speculate, but they have to work the way the Ministry of Health demands from them."

It is interesting to note that in a similar vein, some of Alex Goldfarb's critics ascribed his successes to the fact that he brought with him the cash of a generous donor—George Soros—and "bought" support. Questions were raised, and are still being raised, about whether his projects could continue once the major donor's support ended. Would support be found from other sources? From the government? Program directors like Goldfarb usually go to great lengths to try to incorporate local involvement and leadership to sustain the program, but when donors have left, the sustainability of the program has often been disappointing.

Russian lung experts and politicians wanted to keep their own "rich expertise." They swore that TB in Russia was different from TB elsewhere.

Everybody who works in TB internationally has heard that tale before. Experts in every country begin by saying, "Our TB is different. You don't understand our problem." After much huffing and puffing, arguing and memo writing, usually rational people finally come to a conference table and realize that TB is the same everywhere. But Russian experts hadn't come to that realization yet. TB was the same in Russia as everywhere else; Russia just had the world's worst epidemic of multi-drug-resistant TB. Perhaps for no reason other than pure nationalism—I call it "medical jingoism"—Russian and international experts had not reached a consensus on the treatment of TB in Russia. Western-oriented experts like those at the Khomenko institute supported the approach of the World Health Organization, while other Russian experts wanted to continue with the old Russian system, even enhancing and rebuilding it when necessary. A consensus of TB experts was needed before the political will to support the program could be achieved.

Concerned about the lack of progress that may have been holding up the loan, Goldfarb, Farmer, and I wrote to the minister of health, pointing out the inadequacy of the traditional Russian methods, which contradicted World Health Organization guidelines. Only the first method—basically the World Health Organization's approach supported by the Khomenko institute—met international standards. The other methods of treatment would harm patients and promote drug resistance, and were unacceptable to the international TB community. The ministry's response was curt: We were told that the third set of recommendations, the traditional method, was official government policy and that Russian doctors had a *legal responsibility to follow it*.

Goldfarb was outspoken, as usual. If the Russian authorities didn't follow the universally accepted WHO approach endorsed by the Khomenko institute, he would quit and ask his partners in the PHRI/Soros operation to end the Russian TB program (including the program in Tomsk) because the approach of the ministry would actually be harmful to patients.

By this time, October 2000, Goldfarb had been working flat out on tuberculosis for 5 years. He had suffered a major disappointment when the Gates Foundation had turned down his request for funding of the PHRI's Russian TB project at the time it gave $46 million to Harvard's Paul Farmer and Jim Kim's Partners in Health for treatment of MDR-TB in Peru.

Even before that disappointment, Goldfarb had been showing signs that he was getting bored and wanted to move on to something else—perhaps his old interest in human rights, or even Russian politics, going back to his

student days at Moscow University. Goldfarb remained mercurial, impetu-
ous, stubborn, and very well connected. He was neither a classical academic
scientist nor a typical paper-pushing bureaucrat, so scientists, academics, and
bureaucrats did not know how to deal with him. Inadvertently but invariably, he often offended all of them, while managing to achieve successes they
never could, thanks to his impulsive style, his connections, and his skills in
negotiation.

Reflecting his uncanny ability to get things done effectively while at the
same time upsetting the applecart, by the autumn of 2000, Goldfarb had
fallen out with his major benefactor George Soros, fallen in with the Russian
oligarch Boris Berezovsky, rescued a former Russian spy from Turkey, found
the spy asylum in Great Britain, and got himself on the blacklist of the British
Foreign Office and, perhaps, of the Russian authorities.

In the autumn of 2000, Goldfarb announced that he was officially
resigning as director of the Public Health Research Institute's program in
Russia, effective March 2001—only a few months away.

Soros had already signaled that he was getting ready to pull out of his
public health work to combat TB. He felt that he had made his most important contribution in getting the program started, supporting it, and giving
Goldfarb a platform, and getting other interest and involvement from new
players. He felt that now it was time for other people to take over. He was
committed to support the PHRI program to its completion in a few years,
but made it quite clear that he expected the World Bank loan to take over
when he left. If there was to be no loan, he would certainly not feel oblig-
ated to continue.

The oligarch Berezovsky was an old colleague of Goldfarb's as well as
the sworn enemy of Russian President Vladimir Putin. Goldfarb, probably
at Berezovsky's urging, perhaps in an effort to embarrass Putin, had started
a fund for the families of the men who had been killed in the Kursk submarine disaster in the summer of 2000. A very large contribution came from
Berezovsky himself.

At the same time—the autumn of 2000—Goldfarb was discussing a new
project with Berezovsky: the International Foundation for Civil Liberties.
Berezovsky pledged $25 million and set up the headquarters of the nonprofit
foundation in New York. He is chairman of the board; Goldfarb is vice president. "It fits in very well with his argument with Putin; the oligarch versus
the dictator," Goldfarb explains.

Perhaps Berezovsky saw the Foundation as part of his conflict with
Putin. Berezovsky had made millions from the privatization of the Soviet
state enterprises.[4] He had started as a major supporter of Putin, but after

they became enemies, Berezovsky fled to a luxurious villa in Cap d'Antibes on the French Riviera.

Spy Story

One of Berezovsky's colleagues, according to Goldfarb, had been the spy Alexander Litvinenko. Litvinenko had been a colonel in the Russian FSB, the federal security service that is a successor to the KGB and deals with internal crime. Litvinenko had revealed an FSB plot to kill Berezovsky. Berezovsky had employed and had been able to protect him after he left the FSB, but by 2001 Berezovsky had broken with Putin, had lost political influence, and was hiding out in France.

Fearing for their lives, Litvinenko and his wife and son fled to Turkey, one of the few countries that Russians can enter without a visa. Goldfarb showed up in Turkey, probably at Berezovsky's urging, and escorted the Litvinenkos to the U.S. embassy in Ankara to ask for asylum. U.S. officials, uncertain about result of the coming November 2000 presidential election, suggested that they return in a few weeks.

The Litvinenkos were terrified. Goldfarb bought them airline tickets via London to Barbados, which Russians could also enter without a visa. In the transit lounge of London's Heathrow airport, they ripped up and flushed away their onward tickets. Goldfarb called the lawyer who had represented him years before when he had been arrested at Heathrow for carrying a pocket knife received as a gift (another legendary Goldfarb story) and explained that the Litvinenkos wanted to apply for political asylum. The Litvinenkos were released in custody of the lawyer while their plea for asylum was considered. The story hit both the British papers and the international press. Goldfarb said that the Litvinenkos are still living in London on money lent by Berezovsky and had finally been granted asylum.

As for Goldfarb, the British immigration authorities "told me to get on the first plane and get out." Since then, he has been barred from entry into Britain for the offense of facilitating the entry of an undocumented alien. He has not tested his popularity in Russia, but at least during the Putin administration he is likely to be unwelcome.

New Players

With Goldfarb soon to be out of the picture, Soros's Open Society Institute and PHRI began negotiating with Paul Farmer and Jim Kim's Partners in Health to take over the Tomsk program, for which their group had been serving as medical consultants. They knew it well, and they had a good DOTS-Plus team that had learned and enhanced its skills in Peru. Thus, they could get into action quickly. The Soros funding would continue for two more years. Even though never openly stated, PHRI hoped that perhaps some of Gates's $46 million for Peru could be used in Tomsk.

The major change was that Farmer and Kim would have to begin to deal with the argumentative parties who were negotiating the rules for the World Bank loan. The World Health Organization negotiators who were assisting the World Bank people had already agreed to drop the term *DOTS*. This term had greatly offended the Russians, for reasons that were never clear. Some Russians said that DOTS was a dirty word in Russian or was unlucky; others said that it translated as "the bare minimum of care," which no patient would want. WHO agreed to drop the term, but not the principles of DOTS and DOTS-Plus.

Farmer had an especially delicate role to play. He is passionate, but he also has the friendly skills of a diplomat. He knew from his experience in Lima, Peru, that Russia needed two supportive programs: standard DOTS to treat patients with ordinary TB, and DOTS-Plus to treat patients with multi-drug-resistant TB. The patients with multi-drug-resistant TB would need drug-sensitivity testing followed by individualized treatment with the drugs to which their TB bugs were sensitive, as successfully demonstrated in Peru. In meetings he soothed Russian rage against the Western approach and seemed amenable to blending the two approaches whenever possible. "No hassle. We're friends trying to do a good job curing people" seemed to be his message.

In an interview with *Time* magazine,[5] he said, "Many of our Russian colleagues argued years ago that current international recommendations, which called for all newly diagnosed TB cases to receive exactly the same drugs at the same doses, would not work in Russia. International experts called the Russians misguided and out of date, but time has proven the Russians correct on that score, largely because patients with drug-resistant TB will not respond to treatment with the very drugs to which their infecting strains are resistant."

Farmer was absolutely right: Because there was *already* so much multi-drug-resistant TB in Russia, the ideal would be to do drug-resistance testing on each patient and then treat the patient with the drugs to which he or she was not resistant. Unfortunately, Russia didn't have the laboratory capabilities to do that. DOTS-Plus requires laboratories that can identify strains of multi-drug-resistant TB and do drug-sensitivity testing. Without them, DOTS-Plus cannot be used effectively.

But Farmer also said that there was no need to hospitalize patients for long periods, as Russian doctors did. In Haiti's central plateau, which he called "a God-forsaken hellhole," Farmer's group seldom hospitalized TB patients. The patients did well with treatment at home. In fact, Farmer said, cure rates among poor peasants in Haiti were 95 to 100 percent, compared to 46 percent in Russia. Outpatient care for TB is the standard of care in most programs around the world.

However, the "old Russian patriotic school," as Goldfarb called it, took a different view of Farmer's carefully worded, conciliatory approach. They presented Farmer's views as actually *supporting* the traditional Russian practice of individualizing treatment for each patient, giving whatever drugs and dosages the doctor felt like, without bacteriological confirmation of the patient's drug-sensitivity profile. It was just this approach that had led to the development of multi-drug-resistant TB and created the present problem.

Fran DuMelle of the American Lung Association could have explained that even with careful wording, Russian policy makers would never understand the difference between Farmer's approach and the traditional Russian approach. After all, the policy makers and negotiators were politicians and lawyers, not doctors and public health people. Probably they would remain confused and so would be inclined to do nothing.

What was needed was an international consensus of public health leaders and doctors on following evidence-based medical principles. They had to agree on what needed to be done and the best way to do it, and then send the message to the policy makers. We hoped that such a consensus was being developed in the long negotiations between the World Bank, the World Health Organization, and the Russian Ministries of Health and Justice. Alas, each side still seemed to have its own interpretation, and there still was no consensus when Goldfarb prepared to hand over control of the Tomsk program to Farmer and Kim.

Russian public health officials and Russian doctors had a lot to lose if their entrenched system of X-rays, long hospitalizations, and frequent surgery was overthrown without a new system being put in place that would keep them employed and paid, and their families fed. Doctors were paid by the number of occupied beds in their hospitals. If many doctors and hospital beds were replaced by nurses and outpatient workers, there would be major economic and social disruption. In trying to move the Russian system toward a more efficient, lower-cost method of treating TB that worked in the West and in many Third World countries, Farmer and Kim had delicate roles to play. They needed to be sensitive to the very real needs of Russian health-care workers and responsive to the concerns voiced by Perelman, who did not want to see the old Soviet system destroyed, however clunky it was. The skills of its doctors, technicians, and nurses should not be lost. These skills should be transferred to a better, more efficient, and cost-effective system that would actually be easier for patients.

The Loan, Again

Maybe it was the overwhelming desire for progress and movement, but it actually seemed that the loan agreement with the World Bank had been finally agreed on in the early spring of 2001, although it had not been officially signed and consensus on treatment guidelines still had not been achieved.

Off the record, senior WHO officials insisted to me that if the loan was accepted, payments would be made in several steps and would require the Russians to follow international standards of treating TB or else the money would stop. I hoped they were right, but I recalled Perelman's words on two separate occasions: "We will tell them whatever they want to hear, but when we get the money, we'll spend it as we please." I suspected this was not likely to be in accordance with Western evidence-based guidelines.

A consensus on effective treatment of Russia's epidemic of TB and multi-drug-resistant TB would have a major beneficial effect on world health. With luck, it would save us from a worldwide disaster of multi-drug-resistant tuberculosis or, even worse, from pan-resistant tuberculosis, the superbug that nothing can cure and that spreads through the air.

Armageddon

In June, the Russian government turned down the loan.

I was stunned. The grim news was best told in a story by Andrew Jack of the *Financial Times:* "The Russian government has blocked a $150 million World Bank loan for the treatment of tuberculosis and AIDS, triggering fears of a collapse in health funding within the country at a time of growing concern over a TB epidemic and an increase in HIV infection. The loan, which was requested by the Russian government, has been unexpectedly stalled by the Ministry of Health in a clash over treatment methods and World Bank demands for an international competitive tender for TB drugs."[6]

The implications for world health were disastrous. The article quoted Julian Schweitzer, head of the World Bank's Moscow office, as being "not optimistic" that the dispute could be resolved. He estimated that the spread of TB and AIDS would cut the Russian gross domestic product by *1.5 to 2 percent* by 2005! Rejection of the loan meant that international donors would not come up with matching funds and many might pull out of Russia entirely, leaving pilot programs such as the PHRI/MERLIN program in Tomsk without any funds at all.

It was remarkable that the *Financial Times*, an international business newspaper, did the best report on the failed loan. Money talks. The failed loan surely had implications for the health of Russia's workers, and, ominously, for her economy.

Just days later, in mid-June of 2001, I was attending a "think-tank" meeting that has been organized each of the past 7 years by the Royal Netherlands Tuberculosis Association (KNCV) to discuss tuberculosis in Europe, Eastern Europe, and the former Soviet Union. The Dutch were clever: They isolated us in a comfortable inn in the small town of Wolfheze with good food and drink and very difficult transportation. There was no way participants could make a speech and scoot out to the delights of Amsterdam or The Hague. All of us—more than 100 delegates and observers from 52 countries—would admire the attractive woods through the conference hall windows, and listen to, meet with, and share insights with participants from Europe, Eastern Europe, the former Soviet Union, and also countries in the Middle East, the Far East, Africa, the Indian subcontinent, and Australia. This wasn't a "listen to the speeches and go home" meeting. After we listened, we spent the rest of the day thrashing out the best way to deal with problems: migration, both legal and illegal, of people who might be infected with TB, including asylum seekers; the spread of HIV/AIDS and its connection with TB; the best way to find TB cases (surveillance); DNA fingerprinting to find clusters of TB cases; and the role of TB screening in disaster relief in areas such as the Balkans and Chechnya in Russia. It was a scientifically rigorous and fascinating exchange among doctors, scientists, and public health people. Simultaneous translation was provided for the Russian speakers.

Then Professor Margarita Victorovna Shilova, deputy director of the department for epidemiology and organization for TB control and deputy director for science of the Research Institute of Phthisiopulmonogy of the Moscow Medical Academy of the Ministry of Health, gave her talk about TB in Russia. The audience was polite but flabbergasted. She said that reports of the TB problem in Russia were misleading. Official TB rates now included prisoners with TB, which she felt was a mistake. There was no Russian TB problem, if one did not include the TB cases in the prisons. As if prisoners were not part of the population! As if they were not now infecting their fellow prisoners and the prison staff! As if they would not take their disease home! Furthermore, Shilova said, there is no need for international funding to defeat a Russian TB epidemic that, she said, didn't exist. Russia had the funds and resources to deal with the situation.

Jaws dropped. Heads shook. People rolled their eyes in amazement. Later, we talked about it in the bar, but being polite, nobody raised the question with Shilova, who had retired with the other Russians. We wondered: Why did the Russians ask for a World Bank loan to combat their epidemic, which the experts in the audience had heard about for years, and now the Russians claimed not to have an epidemic at all? Of course, President Putin was said to be opposed to Russia seeking international loans and the government had lately begun to make it difficult for Russian scientists to maintain international contacts.

I recalled very well that highly respected Russian TB professors, such as Alexey Primak, Mikhail Perelman, and Aivar Strelis, had all told Janice in separate interviews that during Soviet times one of their biggest problems and embarrassments as scientists had been that tuberculosis rates were a *state secret*. No one knew the true TB rate, but it had to be reported as going down every year.

Shilova's report sounded, at least to me, shockingly like the same old Soviet story: Everything's fine. Things are getting better. We can take care of it. We will report the numbers you would like to hear.

Epilogue
The Kursk Syndrome

When we set out to write this book, the world faced an impending tuberculosis disaster—more cases than ever, more deaths, and an epidemic raging out of control in tandem with AIDS.

But there were major reasons to hope we could control and eventually conquer TB and multi-drug-resistant TB. Many promising approaches were coming together.

Stop TB, a joint initiative of the World Health Organization and more than 100 partners, emerged as a true, functional partnership with new, enlightened leadership.

New, talented, enthusiastic "unusual suspects" were getting involved in TB. They brought unprecedented amounts of political will and changed the way people saw the disease. For the first time, tuberculosis was considered as an economic handicap, a tourism problem, or a matter of national defense, rather than a social problem. Donations and involvement from major foundations were hopeful signs. DOTS was accepted by 128 countries and efforts were under way to expand its use to all TB patients in a nation. Research efforts were seeking new drugs and vaccines. The new Global Drug Facility was set up to provide effective, high-quality drugs at low cost to nations that needed them.

Even though Russia appeared the lone holdout for adopting up-to-date, proven, evidence-based treatments for TB, we were hopeful that despite her nationalism and stubbornness, she would ultimately join the global community in sincere, joint efforts to control TB. The World Bank loan, so long and carefully negotiated with advice from the World Health Organization, would actually enable Russia to adopt the international standard for treating TB and to incorporate it into its old, disintegrating TB treatment system, while "saving face" if necessary.

All these positive approaches, we thought, would lead to the happy ending that we had hoped for when we set out to write this book.

Alas, there is no happy ending.

I was stunned when the Russian government rejected the World Bank loan in June 2001. The rejection meant that Russia would not be able to get the assistance it needs to begin to fix its disastrous tuberculosis problem, which is already spreading to the West. Just as serious was the fact that the rejection would likely mean the end to matching funds from international donor organizations for treating Russia's TB and HIV/AIDS epidemic.

Why did the Russian government reject the World Bank loan?

I suspect that it is what I call the "Kursk syndrome." When the Russian nuclear submarine Kursk sank on August 12, 2000, the Russians rejected repeated foreign offers to help rescue sailors who might still be alive. When Norwegian and British divers finally were allowed to assist and opened the escape hatch a week later, all the crew were dead. During the unspeakable hours waiting for rescue that never came, two crew members had written messages that rescuers found on their bodies.

The tragic Kursk story may teach us something. The real reason Russia rejected the World Bank loan is national pride: the same reason that Russia rejected help to save the Kursk sailors. National pride comes ahead of individual lives.

Our previous hopeful outcome is now uncertain. Because of Russian medical jingoism, tuberculosis and multi-drug-resistant TB are a present and rapidly increasing risk to the citizens of Russia, and to all of us who live in the world and breathe its air. TB doesn't stay at home. It spreads through the air, and you get it by breathing. Diseases travel with people, and never has it been easier and faster to travel. No place on Earth is more than 24 hours away from another. As John Donne said 400 years ago: "No man is an island."

Notes

Preface

1. T. R. Frieden, P. I. Fujiwara, R. M. Washko, and M. A. Hamburg, "Tuberculosis in New York City—Turning the Tide," *New England Journal of Medicine* 333: 229–233, 1995.
2. World Health Organization, press release, March 22, 2001.
3. S. Sachs, "A Hue, and a Cry, In the Heartland," *New York Times*, Week in Review, April 8, 2001, p. 5.

Chapter 1

1. Public health authorities depend on confidentiality when they investigate disease outbreaks. Without it, individuals, companies, and communities would refuse to help, and the public would be at great risk. Therefore, we cannot identify the airline or many of the participants involved in this case of drug-resistant tuberculosis imported from the former Soviet Union. Individuals who are named gave us their consent.
2. P. E. Farmer, A. F. Kononets, S. E. Borisov, et al., "Recrudescent Tuberculosis in the Russian Federation," in P. Farmer and J. Kim, eds., *The Global Impact of Drug-Resistant Tuberculosis*, Program in Infectious Disease and Social Change, Department of Social Medicine, Harvard Medical School, Harvard Medical School/Open Society Institute, Boston, 1999, pp. 63, app. 4–45.
3. P. Tribble, *TB Notes 2000* 1, U.S. Department of Health and Human Services, Centers for Disease Control, 2000, pp. 68–70.
4. "News in Brief: W.H.O. Warning for Air Passengers," *Lancet* 353: 305, 1999.
5. T. A. Kenyon, S. E. Valway, W. W. Ihle, et al., "Transmission of Multidrug-Resistant *Mycobacterium tuberculosis* during a Long Airplane Flight," *New England Journal of Medicine* 334: 933–938, 1996.
6. R. Marini, "Breathing Easy: Are Proposed New Standards for Air Quality in Passenger Cabins Too Low?" *Frequent Flyer*, March 2000, pp. 20–25.
7. Personal communication from Martha Waters, Ph.D., Senior Researcher with the National Institute for Occupational Safety and Health, Cincinnati, Ohio, March 5, 2001.

Chapter 2

1. J. Grosset, C. Truffot-Pernod, and E. Cambau, "The Bacteriology of Tuberculosis," in L. B. Reichman and E. S. Hershfield, eds., *Tuberculosis: A Comprehensive International Approach*, Marcel Dekker, Inc., New York, 2000, pp. 165–168.
2. D. Satcher, "Tuberculosis—Battling an Ancient Scourge," *JAMA* 282: 1996, 1999.
3. *Dorland's Illustrated Medical Dictionary*, 29th ed., W. B. Saunders Company, Philadelphia, 2000, p. 1384.
4. E. A. Nardell and W. F. Piessens, "Transmission of Tuberculosis," in Reichman and Hershfield, eds., *Tuberculosis*, p. 226.
5. H. Rolleston, "Samuel Johnson's Medical Experiences," in A. Sorsby, ed., *Tenements of Clay*, Charles Scribner's Sons, New York, 1974, p. 142.
6. D. Green, *Queen Anne*, Charles Scribner's Sons, New York, 1970, p. 105.
7. W. H. McNeill, *Plagues and People*, Anchor Press/Doubleday, Garden City, NY, 1976, p. 177.
8. G. M. Trevelyan, *English Social History*, Pelican/Penguin Books Ltd., Harmondsworth, Middlesex, Eng., 1977, pp. 306, 358.
9. D. Cruickshank and P. Wyld, *London: The Art of Georgian Building*, The Architectural Press Ltd., London, 1982, p. 169.
10. T. Dormandy, *The White Death*, New York University Press, New York, 2000, p. 79.
11. Loc. cit.
12. There is no clear numerical definition of epidemic; it means an outbreak of disease in which there are many more cases than usual. The word comes from a Greek word meaning "upon the people."
13. T. M. Daniel, *Captain of Death: The Story of Tuberculosis*, University of Rochester Press, 1997, p. 27.
14. Loc. cit.
15. Ibid., p. 30.
16. S. M. Rothman, *Living in the Shadow of Death*, Johns Hopkins University Press, Baltimore, 1995, p. 2.
17. Committee on the Elimination of Tuberculosis in the United States, Division of Health Promotion and Disease Prevention, Institute of Medicine, *Ending Neglect: The Elimination of Tuberculosis in the United States*, L. Geiter, ed., National Academy Press, Washington, DC, 2000, pp. 23–27.
18. J. T. Flexner, *George Washington: The Forge of Experience (1732–1775)*, Little, Brown and Company, Boston, 1965, p. 49.
19. Ibid., pp. 51, 184, 186, 209, 221–222, 237–238.
20. Daniel, *Captain of Death*, p. 104 (quoting biographies of Keats).
21. Ibid., pp. 101–106.
22. Ibid., pp. 31–32.
23. R. Dubos and J. Dubos, *The White Plague: Tuberculosis, Man, and Society*, Rutgers University Press, New Brunswick, NJ, 1996, pp. 86–87.
24. D. N. Evans, "A Visit to Thomas Wakley," *Lancet* 342: 1535–1536, 1993.
25. B. Lerner, "The Death of Eleanor Roosevelt: Missed Diagnosis or Inevitable Outcome?" *Washington Post*, Health Section, February 2, 2000.
26. Loc. cit.
27. Dubos and Dubos, *The White Plague*, pp. 178–179.

28. Daniel, *Captain of Death*, pp. 186–187.
29. A. L. Davis, "A Historical Perspective on Tuberculosis and Its Control," in Reichman and Hershfield, eds., *Tuberculosis*, p. 25.

Chapter 3

1. The general discussion of Koch's work is drawn from the following sources: T. M. Daniel, *Captain of Death: The Story of Tuberculosis*, University of Rochester Press, 1997, pp. 74–86; R. Dubos and J. Dubos, *The White Plague: Tuberculosis, Man, and Society*, Rutgers University Press, New Brunswick, NJ, 1996, p. 101; T. Dormandy, *The White Death*, New York University Press, 2000, pp. 127–137; and F. Ryan, *The Forgotten Plague: How the Battle against Tuberculosis Was Won and Lost*, Back Bay Books/Little, Brown and Company, Boston, 1992, pp. 9–17.
2. R. Koch, "The Aetiology of Tuberculosis," in *Source Book of Medical History*, compiled with notes by L. Clendening, Dover Publications, Inc., New York, 1960, pp. 392–406 (republication of 1942 edition).
3. C. Tomiche and F. Tomiche, "One Hundred Years Ago—Koch's Bacillus" (two-page press backgrounder), International Union against Tuberculosis and World Health Organization, March 24, 1982.
4. "Postulate," in *Dorland's Illustrated Medical Dictionary*, 29th ed., W. B. Saunders Company, Philadelphia, 2000.
5. The source for much of the following historical discussion is A. L. Davis, "A Historical Perspective on Tuberculosis and Its Control," in L. B. Reichman and E. S. Hershfield, eds., *Tuberculosis: A Comprehensive International Approach*, Marcel Dekker, Inc., New York, 2000, pp. 3–54.
6. V. N. Houk, "Spread of Tuberculosis Via Recirculated Air in a Naval Vessel: The Byrd Study," *Annals of the New York Academy of Sciences* 353: 10–24, 1980.
7. Davis, "Historical Perspective," p. 19.
8. Ibid.
9. There are a few other acid-fast bacteria in the same family as *Mycobacterium tuberculosis*, so while a positive acid-fast smear is strongly suggestive, it is not absolute proof that the person has TB.
10. Daniel, *Captain of Death*, pp. 196–197.
11. Davis, "Historical Perspective," p. 33.
12. The term *vaccination* comes from *vaccinia*, the Latin name for cowpox, which in turn is derived from the Latin word *vacca*, or cow.
13. L. Pasteur, "Prevention of Rabies," in *Source Book of Medical History*, compiled with notes by L. Clendening, Dover Publications, Inc., New York, 1960, pp. 388–392 (republication of 1942 edition).
14. Daniel, *Captain of Death*, pp. 114, 171.
15. Koch, "Aetiology of Tuberculosis," pp. 392–406; also Daniel, *Captain of Death*, pp. 82–84.
16. Daniel, *Captain of Death*, pp. 83–84; Dubos and Dubos, *The White Plague*, pp. 107–110.
17. Daniel, *Captain of Death*, p. 174.
18. Davis, "Historical Perspective," p. 33.
19. Daniel, *Captain of Death*, p. 174.
20. Davis, "Historical Perspective," p. 34.

21. Loc. cit.; another test that is still sometimes used employs an applicator with four prickly needles; called the Tine test, it is inaccurate because it is impossible to determine the amount of tuberculin on the needles or how deeply they have been inserted into the skin.
22. Daniel, *Captain of Death*, pp. 134–142.
23. Davis, "Historical Perspective," p. 36.
24. Daniel, *Captain of Death*, p. 136.
25. Davis, "Historical Perspective," pp. 36–37.
26. G. W. Comstock, "Field Trials of Tuberculosis Vaccines: How Could We Have Done Them Better?" *Controlled Clinical Trials* 15: 247–276, 1994.
27. P. E. M. Fine, "BCG Vaccines and Vaccination," in L. B. Reichman and E. S. Hershfield, eds.,*Tuberculosis*, pp. 504–522.
28. M. A. Brower, K. M. Edwards, P. S. Palmer, et al., "Bacille Calmette Guérin Immunization in Normal Healthy Adults," *Journal of Infectious Diseases* 170: 476–479, 1994.
29. "The Role of BCG Vaccine in the Prevention and Control of Tuberculosis in the United States: A Joint Statement by the Advisory Council for the Elimination of Tuberculosis and the Advisory Committee on Immunization Practices," *Morbidity and Mortality Weekly Report* 45 (no. RR-4), 1–18, 1996.
30. T. V. Lyagoshina, "Russia," in P. D. O. Davies, ed., *Clinical Tuberculosis*, Chapman & Hall, London, 1998.
31. D. L. Heymann, A. Kochi, and M. C. Raviglione, "Foreword," in P. Farmer and J. Kim, eds., *The Global Impact of Drug-Resistant Tuberculosis*, Program in Infectious Disease and Social Change, Department of Social Medicine, Harvard Medical School, Harvard Medical School/Open Society Institute, Boston, 1999, p. i.
32. The following paragraphs are based on Daniel, *Captain of Death*, pp. 204–214.
33. Ibid., p. 207; "Researcher's Family Says She Deserved More Credit for Drug" (obituary for Elizabeth Bugie Gregory), *The Record*, Hackensack, NJ, April15, 2001.
34. An additional source for this and the following paragraph is Dormandy, *The White Death*, pp. 364–366.

Chapter 4

1. G. Sunderam, T. Maniatis, R. Kapila, et al., "*Mycobacterium tuberculosis* with Unusual Manifestations Is Relatively Common in Acquired Immunodeficiency Syndrome (AIDS)," *American Review of Respiratory Diseases* 129(suppl.): 191, 1984.
2. L. B. Reichman, C. P. Felton, and J. Edsall, "Drug Dependence: A New Risk Factor for Tuberculosis Disease," *Archives of Internal Medicine* 139: 337–339, 1979.
3. G. Sunderam, R. J. McDonald, T. Maniatis, et al., "Tuberculosis as a Manifestation of the Acquired Immunodeficiency Syndrome (AIDS)," *JAMA* 256: 362–366, 1986.
4. E. Bishburg, G. Sunderam, L. B. Reichman, and R. Kapila, "Central Nervous System Tuberculosis with the Acquired Immunodeficiency Syndrome and Its Related Complex," *Annals of Internal Medicine* 105: 210–213, 1986.
5. L. B. Reichman, "HIV Infection—A New Face of Tuberculosis," *Bulletin of the International Union against Tuberculosis and Lung Disease* 63 (no. 3): 19–26, 1988.
6. R. D. McFadden, "A Drug-Resistant TB Results in 13 Deaths in New York Prisons," *New York Times*, November 16, 1991, A1, A22.

7. Loc. cit.

8. R. D. McFadden, "Rare TB Strain Kills 13th Inmate in New York Prisons," *New York Times,* Nov. 17, 1991, A39.

9. "AIDS Epidemic Update," UNAIDS, Geneva, Switzerland, December 1999.

10. K. M. DeCock, B. Soro, I. M. Coulibaly, and S. B. Lucas, "Tuberculosis and HIV Infection in Sub-Saharan Africa," *JAMA* 268: 1581–1587, 1992.

11. F. C. Notzon, Y. M. Komarov, S. P. Ermakov, et al., "Causes of Declining Life Expectancy in Russia," *JAMA* 279: 793–800, 1998.

12. Telephone interview with Masha Gessen, journalist with *Itogi* (Russian newsweekly affiliated with *Newsweek*), February 22, 2000.

13. I. Danilova, L. Mitunina, M. Urastova, et al., "Tuberculosis Treatment Interruptions—Ivanovo Oblast, Russian Federation, 1999," *Morbidity and Mortality Weekly Report,* Centers for Disease Control and Prevention, Atlanta, March 23, 2001, 50 (11): 201–204.

14. M. Feshbach, "A Sick and Shrinking Nation," *Washington Post,* October 24, 1999, B07.

15. P. E. Farmer, A. F. Kononets, S. E. Borisov, et al., "Recrudescent Tuberculosis in the Russian Federation," in P. Farmer and J. Kim, eds., *The Global Impact of Drug-Resistant Tuberculosis,* Program in Infectious Disease and Social Change, Department of Social Medicine, Harvard Medical School, Harvard Medical School/Open Society Institute, Boston, 1999, p. 46.

16. Ibid., pp. 47–49, 51.

17. "Facts and Figures," in V. Stern, ed., *Sentenced to Die? The Problem of TB in Prisons in Eastern Europe and Central Asia,* International Centre for Prison Studies, King's College, London, 1999, p. 42.

18. Farmer, Kononets, Borisov, et al., "Recrudescent Tuberculosis," pp. 52–60.

19. Ibid., p. 52.

20. Ibid., p. 59.

21. M. Wines, "Heroin Carries AIDS to a Region in Siberia," *New York Times,* April 24, 2000, A1, A12.

22. Feshbach, "A Sick and Shrinking Nation," B07.

23. Wines, "Heroin Carries AIDS," A1, A12.

24. M. Wines, "Needle Use Sets Off HIV Explosion in Russia," *New York Times,* November 24, 1999.

25. O. Yablokova, "Russia Says It Is Trying to Head Off AIDS Epidemic," *Moscow Times,* November 30, 1999.

26. "AIDS Epidemic Update," Report of the Joint United Nations Program on HIV/AIDS (UNAIDS) and the World Health Organization (WHO), December 1999.

27. J. Hendren, "Loans Help Couples Afford Adoption," *New York Times,* (Sunday Business Section), February 18, 2000, BU11.

Chapter 5

1. "On Approval of Standards (Model Protocols) of Tuberculosis Patient Management," Prikaz 33 (Order 33), Ministry of Health of the Russian Federation, Moscow, February 2, 1998.

2. D. L. Heymann, A. Kochi, and M. C. Raviglione, "Foreword," in P. Farmer and J. Kim, eds., *The Global Impact of Drug-Resistant Tuberculosis*, Program in Infectious Disease and Social Change, Department of Social Medicine, Harvard Medical School, Harvard Medical School/Open Society Institute, Boston, 1999, p.i.
3. P. E. Farmer, A. F. Kononets, S. E. Borisov, et al., "Recrudescent Tuberculosis in the Russian Federation,"in P. Farmer and J. Kim, eds., *The Global Impact*, pp. 61–62.
4. D. G. McNeil, Jr., "Resisting Drugs, TB Spreads Fast in the West," *New York Times*, March 24, 2000.
5. A. C. Hayward and R. J. Coker, "Could a Tuberculosis Epidemic Occur in London as It Did in New York?" *Emerging Infectious Diseases* 6, www.cdc.gov/nci-dod/eid/vol6no1/ascii/hayward.txt, 2000.
6. J. Miller, "Study Says New TB Strains Need an Intensive Strategy," *New York Times*, October 28, 1999, A6.

Chapter 6

1. S. Chapkovsky and N. Bock, "Case Study of Tuberculosis in the Russian Correctional System," in L. B. Reichman and E. S. Hershfield, eds., *Tuberculosis: A Comprehensive International Approach*, Marcel Dekker, Inc., New York, 2000, App. A, pp. 657–660.
2. Loc. cit.
3. A. Coyle, "Prison Reform and the Management of TB in Eastern Europe and Central Asia," in V. Stern, ed., *Sentenced to Die? The Problem of TB in Prisons in Eastern Europe and Central Asia*, International Centre for Prison Studies, King's College, London, 1999, pp. 52–53.
4. P. Farmer, "Cruel and Unusual: Drug-Resistant Tuberculosis as Punishment," in V. Stern, ed., *Sentenced to Die? The Problem of TB in Prisons in Eastern Europe and Central Asia*, International Centre for Prison Studies, King's College, London, 1999, p. 78.
5. A. Goldfarb, "Multi-Drug-Resistant TB in the Former Soviet Union: A Global Threat," summary of presentation at *TB in Eastern Europe* seminar, Salzburg, Austria, January 16–20, 1999.
6. *Moscow Times*, March 25, 2000.
7. P. Henderson, "Russia's Ailing Jails Set for Change, Lack Funds," Reuters, October 15, 1997.
8. C. O'Dea, "Spectre of TB Haunts Russian Jails," *Irish Times*, July 20, 1998.
9. S. Karush, "Thousands Pour into Crowded Prisons," *Moscow Times*, June 1, 1999.
10. A. Stanley, "Jails in Russia: The Crime of Punishment," *New York Times*, January 8, 1998.
11. Coyle, "Prison Reform," p. 61.
12. Chapkovsky and Bock, "Case Study of Tuberculosis," pp. 657–660.
13. "Russia Seeks to Improve Grim Prisons," Reuters, Moscow, April 2, 1999.
14. Stanley, "Jails in Russia."
15. Sir. N. Rodley, quoted in V. Stern "Introduction: An Overview and Some Issues," in V Stern, ed., *Sentenced to Die?*, p. 12.
16. P. E. Farmer, A. F. Kononets, S. E. Borisov, et al., "Recrudescent Tuberculosis in the Russian Federation," in P. Farmer and J. Kim, eds., *The Global Impact of Drug-Resistant Tuberculosis*, Program in Infectious Disease and Social Change,

Department of Social Medicine, Harvard Medical School, Harvard Medical School/Open Society Institute, Boston, 1999, p. 55.

17. Ibid., p. 53.

18. Coyle, "Prison Reform," pp. 57–58.

19. Ibid., pp. 57–60.

20. M. E. Kimerling, H. Kluge, N. Vezhnina, et al., "Inadequacy of the Current WHO Re-Treatment Regimen in a Central Siberian Prison: Treatment Failure and MDR-TB," *International Journal of Tuberculosis and Lung Disease* 3(5): 451–453, 1999.

21. C. Gall, "The Death Stops Here," *Moscow Times*, January 17, 1998; Y. Dlugy, "The Prisoners' Plague," *Newsweek*, July 5, 1999, pp. 18–20.

22. Loc. cit.

23. Kimerling, Kluge, Vezhnina, et al., "Inadequacy of the Current WHO Re-Treatment Regimen."

24. Y. Borisova, "Kemerovo: One Region's TB Profile," *Moscow Times*, January 29, 2000.

25. T. Kidder, "The Good Doctor," *New Yorker*, July 10, 2000, pp. 40–57.

26. The source for this and the following paragraph is M. C. Becerra, J. Bayona, P. E. Farmer, et al., "Defusing a Time Bomb: The Challenge of Antituberculosis Drug Resistance in Peru," in P. Farmer and J. Kim, eds., *The Global Impact*, pp. 109–125.

27. *Russia, Ukraine, and Belarus*, Lonely Planet Publications, Hawthorn (Victoria), Australia, 1996, p. 760.

28. Declaration on the Formation of the Regional Association for the Fight against Tuberculosis, Moscow, September 28, 1999.

29. "The Russian Adventures of Koch's Bacillus," *Novy Izvestiya* (daily newspaper), Moscow, late June or early July 1998, trans. Alex Goldfarb, July 2, 1998.

30. Dr. Mikhail Perelman, personal communication, September 28, 1999.

31. *Report by Program Director Alex Goldfarb*, PHRI/Soros Russian TB Program, Newark, NJ, December 17, 1999.

32. V. A. Krasnov and L. M. Pogozheva, *Reference Note on the Status of Public Anti-TB Services in Tomsk Region*, results of inspection carried out by specialists of the Novosibirsk Research Institute of Tuberculosis (NRIT), April 3–12, 2000, in accordance with Instruction #2510/3008–26 of the Russian Federation Health Ministry, issued March 22, 2000.

33. K. Lambregts-van Weezenbeek, M. Grzemska, and E. Heldal, *TB Control in Tomsk Region: Review by PHRI Advisory Committee*, March 20–25, 2000.

34. P. Farmer, "Drug-Resistant Tuberculosis in Tomsk and Kemerovo Oblasts, Russian Federation, Consultant Report," in P. Farmer and J. Kim, eds., *The Global Impact*, App. 8, p. 3.

Chapter 7

1. *Service Book of the Holy Orthodox Apostolic Church*, revised 5th ed., trans. Isabel Florence Hapgood, Antiochian Orthodox Christian Archdiocese of New York, Englewood, NJ, 1975.

2. T. V. Lyagoshina, "Russia," in P. D. O. Davies, ed., *Clinical Tuberculosis*, Chapman & Hall, London, 1998, pp. 631–642.

3. Ibid., pp. 638–639.

4. F. Drobniewski, E. Tayler, N. Ignatenko, et al., "Tuberculosis in Siberia: 1. An Epidemiological and Microbiological Assessment," in V. Stern, ed., *Sentenced to Die? The Problem of TB in Prisons in Eastern Europe and Central Asia*, International Centre for Prison Studies, King's College, London, 1999, p. 125. (Article reprinted from *Tubercle and Lung Disease* 77: 199–206, 1996.)
5. Ibid., pp. 124–125.
6. Lyagoshina, "Russia," p. 640.
7. F. Drobniewski, E. Tayler, N. Ignatenko, et al, "Tuberculosis in Siberia: 2. Diagnosis, Chemoprophylaxis and Treatment," in V. Stern, ed., *Sentenced to Die?*, p. 140. (Article reprinted from *Tubercle and Lung Disease* 77: 297–301, 1996.)
8. David Ashkin, M.D., State TB Controller, Bureau of Tuberculosis and Refugee Health, Florida Department of Health, personal communication by e-mail, June 14, 2000.
9. P. Farmer and J. Kim, eds., *The Global Impact of Drug-Resistant Tuberculosis*, Program in Infectious Disease and Social Change, Department of Social Medicine, Harvard Medical School, Harvard Medical School/Open Society Institute, Boston, 1999, table, p. 47.
10. I. Danilova, L. Mitunina, M. Urastova, et al., "Tuberculosis Treatment Interruptions—Ivanovo Oblast, Russian Federation, 1999," *Morbidity and Mortality Weekly Report* 50 (no. 11): 201–204, 2001.
11. Interview by JHT with Professor Aivar Karlovich Strelis, Tomsk, October 1, 1999.
12. Masha Gessen, "Tuberculosis: The Triumphant March of Once-Defeated Scourge," *Itogi*, September 16, 1997. English translation provided by the Public Health Research Institute.
13. Interview with Professors Mikhail Perelman and Irine Bogadelnikova, September 28, 1999.
14. V. Stern, "Introduction," in V. Stern, ed., *Sentenced to Die?*, p. 22
15. Interview with Perelman and Bogadelnikova.
16. M. I. Perelman and V. P. Strelzov, "Surgery for Pulmonary Tuberculosis," *World Journal of Surgery* 21: 457–467, 1997.

Chapter 8

1. B. T. Mangura, E. C. Napolitano, M. R. Passannante, et al., "*Mycobacterium tuberculosis* Miniepidemic in a Church Gospel Choir," *Chest* 113: 234–237, 1998.
2. S. E. Valway, M. P. Sanchez, T. F. Shinnick, et al., "An Outbreak Involving Extensive Transmission of a Virulent Strain of *Mycobacterium tuberculosis*," *New England Journal of Medicine* 338: 633–639, 1998.
3. Loc. cit.

Chapter 9

1. D. Remnick, "More Bad News from the Gulag," *New Yorker*, February 15, 1999.
2. *Health of the City: Focus on Tuberculosis*, New York City Department of Health, 1995.
3. T. R. Frieden, P. I. Fujiwara, R. M. Washko, and M. A. Hamburg, "Tuberculosis in New York City—Turning the Tide," *New England Journal of Medicine* 333: 229–233, 1995.

4. Dr. Donna Shalala, U.S. Secretary of Health and Human Services, speaking at the WHO International Tuberculosis Conference, Amsterdam, The Netherlands, March 23, 2000.

5. P. I. Fujiwara, C. Larkin, and T. R. Frieden, "Directly Observed Therapy in New York City: History, Implementation, Results, and Challenges," *Clinics in Chest Medicine* 18: 135–148, 1997; K. Brudney and J. Dobkin, "Resurgent Tuberculosis in New York City," *American Review of Respiratory Disease* 144: 745–749, 1991.

6. Frieden, Fujiwara, Washko, and Hamburg, "Tuberculosis in New York City."

7. T. R. Frieden, T. Sterling, A. Pablos-Mendez, et al., "The Emergence of Drug-Resistant Tuberculosis in New York City," *New England Journal of Medicine* 328: 521–526, 1993.

8. J. Barron, "Panel to Recommend Ways to Fight TB in New York Jails," *New York Times*, June 25, 1992.

9. Fujiwara, Larkin, and Frieden, "Directly Observed Therapy."

Chapter 10

1. L. Belkin, "A Brutal Cure," *New York Times Magazine*, May 30, 1999, pp. 32–39.

Chapter 11

1. L. B. Reichman, "How to Ensure the Continued Resurgence of Tuberculosis," *Lancet* 347: 175–177, 1996.

2. L. K. Altman, "As TB Surges, Drug Producers Face Criticism," *New York Times*, September 18, 1995, A1.

3. S. Chacko, "The Global Market for TB Medicines: Interim Report," in *Proceedings of the Meeting on TB Drug Development*, sponsored by the Rockefeller Foundation, Cape Town, South Africa, February 6–8, 2000.

4. A. Pablos-Mendez and T. C. Evans, "Health Equity and Product Development for Orphan Diseases: Harnessing the New Sciences to Shorten the Treatment of Tuberculosis," in *Proceedings of the Meeting on TB Drug Development*, sponsored by the Rockefeller Foundation, Cape Town, South Africa, February 6–8, 2000.

5. Research on rifapentine is currently being sponsored by the U.S. government's Centers for Disease Control through its Tuberculosis Trials Consortium, which is studying to find the most effective dosage. Within a year or two, I think rifapentine will take its rightful place as the most important part of a 2-month daily intensive treatment program, followed by 4 months of once-a-week treatment. Such a regimen will obviously be easier for the patient as well as for those who provide the treatment.

6. D. Chang-Blanc, "Incentives and Disincentives for New Anti-Tuberculosis Drug Treatment: Situational Analysis," World Health Organization, Geneva (Stop TB position paper presented at Global Research Initiative, Casablanca, Morocco, June 29–July 1, 1999).

7. D. Chang-Blanc and P. Nunn, "Incentives and Disincentives for the Development of New Anti-Tuberculosis Drugs" (revised version of paper cited in ref. 6), in *Proceedings of the Meeting on TB Drug Development*, sponsored by the Rockefeller Foundation, Cape Town, South Africa, February 6–8, 2000.

8. A. Mbewu, "Welcome Remarks," in *Proceedings of the Meeting on TB Drug Development*, sponsored by the Rockefeller Foundation, Cape Town, South Africa, February 6–8, 2000.

9. S. Chacko, "The Global Market for TB Medicines: Interim Report."

10. J. Horton, "Corporate Interest and Corporate Citizenship," in *Proceedings of the Meeting on TB Drug Development*, sponsored by the Rockefeller Foundation, Cape Town, South Africa, February 6–8, 2000.

11. N. Wade, "Scientists Decode the DNA of Germ Responsible for TB," *New York Times*, June 11, 1998, A1.

12. L. Helmuth, "A Weak Link in TB Bacterium Is Found," *Science* 289: 1123–1125, 2000.

13. A. M. Ginsberg, "Tuberculosis Vaccines: State of the Science," from the Web site of the National Institute of Allergy and Infectious Diseases (www.niaid.nih.gov), last updated June 8, 2000.

Chapter 12

1. Institute of Medicine, J. Lederberg, R. E. Shope, and S. C. Oaks, eds., *Emerging Infections*, National Academy Press, Washington, DC, 1992.

2. L. Garrett, *The Coming Plague*, Farrar, Straus & Giroux, New York, 1994.

3. L. Garrett, *Betrayal of Trust*, Hyperion, New York, 2000.

4. "Let the Huddled Masses In," *Economist*, March 31, 2001, p. 15.

5. S. Sachs, "A Hue, and a Cry, in the Heartland," *New York Times*, Week in Review, April 8, 2001, p. 5.

6. C. J. Murray, K. Styblo, and A. Rouillon, "Tuberculosis in Developing Countries: Burden, Intervention, and Cost," *Bulletin of the International Union against Tuberculosis and Lung Disease* 65: 6–24, 1990.

7. The World Bank, *Investing in Health*, Oxford University Press, Washington, DC, 1993.

8. *G8 Communique on Health*, Nago, Okinawa, AP Worldstream, July 23, 2000.

9. Committee on the Elimination of Tuberculosis in the United States, Division of Health Promotion and Disease Prevention, Institute of Medicine, L. Geiter, ed., *Ending Neglect: The Elimination of Tuberculosis in the United States*, National Academy Press, Washington, DC, 2000.

Chapter 13

1. *Meditsinskaya Gazeta (Medical Gazette)*, no. 15, March 2, 2001; translation provided by the Public Health Research Institute.

2. I. Danilova, L. Mitunina, M. Urastova, et al. "Tuberculosis Treatment Interruptions—Ivanovo Oblast, Russian Federation, 1999," *Morbidity and Mortality Weekly Report* 50(11): 201–4, 2001.

3. Alexander Ivanov, "Who Plays Which Tune, or the Way We Are Equated with Africa in TB Control," *Meditsinskaya Gazeta*, no. 39, May 26, 2000. Translation provided by the Public Health Research Institute.

4. Paul Klebnikov, *Godfather of the Kremlin: Boris Berezovsky and the Looting of Russia*. Harcourt, Inc., New York, 2000.

5. Andrew Meier, "The Fight against TB," *Time*, European edition, Time.com, Jan. 16, 2001.

6. Andrew Jack, "Moscow Bars World Bank Loan," *Financial Times*, June 8, 2001.

Hot Zones of MDR-TB

The World Health Organization named the following countries as having a "high burden" of cases of multi-drug-resistant TB in 2001.

Afghanistan
Bangladesh
Brazil
Cambodia
China
Democratic Republic of Congo
Ethiopia
India
Indonesia
Kenya
Mozambique
Myanmar
Nigeria
Pakistan
Philippines
Russia
South Africa
Tanzania
Thailand
Uganda
Vietnam
Zimbabwe

Index

INDEX 237

About the Authors

Lee B. Reichman, M.D., M.P.H. is Executive Director of the New Jersey Medical School National Tuberculosis Center, widely considered to be one of the world's leading TB treatment, training, and research facilities.

Janice Hopkins Tanne is an award-winning medical and science writer whose work has appeared in many magazines, including *New York Magazine*, *Parade*, and *The British Medical Journal*. She lives in New York.